SHAPING CHILDREN'S SERVICES

This text is an authoritative analysis of current services for children and young people in the UK. Drawing upon European-wide data, this innovative book critiques the policies that have shaped today's services, argues that the current system is insufficiently joined-up and outlines a radical new model of co-located services for the integrated delivery of children's care.

Shaping Children's Services:

- examines key indicators of children's development;
- provides a breakdown of the economics of caring for children;
- explores the way government initiatives such as Sure Start, Extended Schools, Total Place and the Kennedy review of children's health have shaped current policies;
- charts the key twentieth-century developments of child welfare across health, education and social care and looks at the inter-relationships between health, social care, police, education and the voluntary sector;
- presents both good and failing examples of children's services.

Offering a thoughtful and provocative challenge on how the present system can be better configured to meet the needs of children and young people, this book is an essential read for all those involved in working with children from a range of fields, including health, education, social care, juvenile justice and voluntary sector services.

Chris Hanvey works as a non-executive director for the NEW Devon Clinical Commissioning Group, with a lead on safeguarding. He was also Vice Chair of the Department of Education's Family Fund and is a Fellow of the RSA and the Dartington Social Policy Unit for children. Until recently, Dr Hanvey was the Chief Executive of the Royal College of Paediatrics and Child Health and, prior to this, was the Deputy CEO of Barnardo's and CEO of the Thomas Coram Foundation.

SHAPING CHILDREN'S SERVICES

Chris Hanvey

Routledge
Taylor & Francis Group
LONDON AND NEW YORK

First published 2019
by Routledge
2 Park Square, Milton Park, Abingdon, Oxon OX14 4RN

and by Routledge
52 Vanderbilt Avenue, New York, NY 10017

Routledge is an imprint of the Taylor & Francis Group, an informa business

British Library Cataloguing-in-Publication Data
A catalogue record for this book is available from the British Library

Library of Congress Cataloging-in-Publication Data
Names: Hanvey, Christopher P., author.
Title: Shaping children's services / Chris Hanvey.
Description: First Edition. | New York : Routledge, 2019. |
Includes bibliographical references and index.
Identifiers: LCCN 2018042343 | ISBN 9780815374626 (hbk) |
ISBN 9780815374640 (pbk) | ISBN 9781351241731 (ebk)
Subjects: LCSH: Social work with children—Great Britain. | Child welfare—Great Britain.
Classification: LCC HV751.A6 H29 2019 | DDC 362.70941—dc23
LC record available at https://lccn.loc.gov/2018042343

ISBN: 978-0-8153-7462-6 (hbk)
ISBN: 978-0-8153-7464-0 (pbk)
ISBN: 978-1-351-24173-1 (ebk)

Typeset in Bembo
by Swales & Willis Ltd, Exeter, Devon, UK

To my family: Rosie, Natasha and Marcus.

CONTENTS

ACKNOWLEDGEMENTS

If it takes a whole village to raise children, it probably takes a city to write about them. I am very grateful to the many city dwellers who over the years have been generously prepared to share their ideas on what a good, integrated service for children might look like. This book has had a much longer gestation than that of an elephant and, on the way, I have been inspired by the numerous views and influence of others.

I would wish to begin with Grace McInnes, at Taylor and Francis, who subtly shaped, encouraged and nurtured an idea, until it was in a fit state to be put to the editorial board. When Grace took maternity leave, to do some integrated child care of her own, I was fortunate to be supported by Charlotte Endersby and Carolina Antunes, both delightful midwives to the book's birth. Also to Rosie Stewart and Ting Baker for their editorial skills and patience.

Apart from our dog, Bracken, who listened to my ideas on long walks but didn't contribute a great deal, I have been enriched by other conversations that did provide encouragement, fresh views and new perspectives. Those who have helped have included Dr Hilary Cass, Professor Norman Tutt, Dr Keith White, Terry Philpot, Dr Bob Jezzard, John Pierson, Dr Tim Hobbs, Dr Ian Maconochie, and Stephen Hanvey. And to Phil Bonser who regularly demonstrates that you can be over 12 years old, still understand computer glitches and patiently put them right.

I am particularly grateful to the Dartington Research Unit and Fellows, orchestrated by the ever insightful and helpful Professor Roger Bullock, who listened to early iterations of the book and made critical, always helpful, comments. There was something particularly moving about sharing ideas in the same elegant room at Dartington Hall where Beveridge, in the darkest days of the Second World War, explored his vision of a welfare state in a world politicians hoped would become very different. It would be good to think that a little of their vision and optimism has permeated some pages of the book.

My career has been spent working with children and I am particularly grateful for the inspiration of Tom White with whom I worked in both Coventry and NCH, and Sir Terence Stephenson, then President of the Royal College of Paediatrics and Child Health. The College was always a source of rich ideas. There was something delightfully unpompous about the place, perhaps because children aren't too impressed by the status of consultants and it rubbed off onto the staff, clinicians and officers who contributed greatly to my thinking. And here I was grateful to have the help of Ravina Khela, a research assistant who quickly grasped the thinking and was indefatigable in the pursuit of research data.

I was also assisted by Hannah Warwick, Principal Officer at NCB, in chasing down material and staff at the Modern Research Centre of Warwick University library.

I owe an unpayable debt to the children and young people with whom I have been privileged to work for over 40 years and who, despite sometimes awful starts to or subsequent events in their lives, were often able to find a resilience and hope that things might just get better.

Lastly, to my family. It is challenging to write a book outlining a vision when the world appears to be imploding on itself. How do you win hearts and minds for a fundamental shift in how we deliver services to the most vulnerable children when the world appears to be turning sharply to the Right, increasingly preoccupied simply with protecting its own and looking no wider than national borders? In this context my family have helped to maintain some optimism. Natasha and Marcus, because they taught me much of what little I know about children and Rosie who has been fundamental both through her encouragement and support and in the production of the book itself. The faults remain solely mine.

FOREWORD

In January 2018, in the 70th anniversary year of the NHS, the Department of Health in England was renamed as the Department of Health and Social Care thus bringing us full circle back to the days of the DHSS – the Department of Health and Social Security between 1968 and 1988, the 20th and 40th anniversaries of the NHS. This is a recognition, at least in name, of what Chris Hanvey's book is all about – that the care of the ill, weak and vulnerable children in society requires a comprehensive and joined-up solution by all the caring professions and organisations, not isolated actions.

Sir Michael Marmot has elegantly shown in a number of groundbreaking reports that the social determinants of health far outweigh the more obvious biological causes of physical and mental illness. Data show that deprivation, measured by income, employment, education, housing and crime, can explain almost half of the variation in male life expectancy at birth between different geographical locations within the UK. Chris Hanvey argues that we need to do more than plug a short-term funding gap in healthcare. By this 70th year of the NHS, public spending on health has gone from 2.5% of GDP in 1953 to 7.4% of GDP but the advances in healthcare, the greater expectations of the public and the improved outcomes and longevity since 1953 mean this is still not enough. We need to rethink the design, delivery and funding of the NHS and social care to meet the needs of our childhood population. Anything short of a system overhaul will almost certainly result in a continued decline in quality of care.

In *Shaping Children's Services*, Chris Hanvey analyses current services for children and young people and looks at the inter-relationships between health, social care, education and the voluntary sector. He charts the key twentieth-century developments of child welfare, across health, education and social care from the consequences of the Boer War, via the onset of Beveridge's Welfare State, to the present diminishing state services and growing voluntary and private sector provision of care.

The book explores the way government initiatives such as Sure Start, Extended Schools, Total Place, the Kennedy review of children's health or the Troubled Families initiative have shaped current policies. It considers good and failing examples of the integration of services and outlines a new model for the delivery of services to children, in order to mend some of the existing fractures.

"Integrated care" is today's zeitgeist but integration can take many forms. Integration between different professions – encapsulated in the multidisciplinary decision-making, which is now fortunately commonplace in paediatric departments within hospitals; vertical integration between secondary care and primary care – recognising that primary care sees 90% of all patients both within office hours and out of hours; horizontal integration between teams in the community – general practitioners, community nursing, community psychiatry, social workers; integrated services built around the child's needs, not the convenience of the professionals delivering those services, leading ideally to a one-stop-shop approach rather than multiple different appointments in multiple different locations; integration between public, private and third sector providers.

Some of these types of integration are well established but others still struggle on the ground. In England, serial attempts to develop an internal market within healthcare over the last three decades, the outsourcing of services to the private sector and the new commissioning arrangements following the 2012 NHS Act have all made integrated working harder. In addition, a period of austerity has resulted in public expenditure on social care for all ages declining by 8% since 2010 as central government has reduced local authority funding, ironically placing an added burden on the NHS. The NHS itself had become used to a year-on-year average increase in real terms funding of around 4% since 1948 but, since 2008, there has been little increase in funding. The organisation of social care remains highly fragmented across local authorities and not integrated with healthcare despite various attempts to do so. The National Audit Office – in an evaluation of two decades of initiatives to integrate health and social care by governments of various persuasions – found "no compelling evidence to show that integration in England leads to sustainable financial savings or reduced hospital activity" (1, p. 7).

Furthermore, we must change the way we think about health more generally – from acute care to prevention. Benjamin Franklin said "an ounce of prevention is worth a pound of cure" and that axiom remains as true today. International comparisons of infant mortality rates show that much of the poorer performance in the UK can be attributed to higher rates of lower birth weight infants born in the UK. This suggests that preventive policies should focus on reducing prenatal risk factors and improving maternal health before and during pregnancy rather than simply increased resources for expensive neonatal intensive care facilities. With approximately a third of British children overweight or obese by the time they transfer from primary school to secondary school and a 15-fold increase over the last decade of type 2 diabetes in young people due to obesity, society needs to tackle the causes of unhealthy lifestyles, not the symptoms. Cleaner air would almost certainly do more to reduce the burden of care from childhood asthma than training more children's doctors and nurses. Governments need to look to the management of population health and the longer-term promotion of wellness and this is grounded in wider economic and social interventions rather than isolated healthcare interventions.

As a practising paediatrician, I write this foreword after another year in which health services for children across the UK are working ever harder and when it is being reported that accident and emergency departments and primary care services are struggling to cope with demand. This challenges our ability as professionals caring for children to provide the high standard of care that we would like to. But it is in these moments – when our skills, compassion and endurance are tested to the limits – that I feel huge pride in the caring professions. Every week I see colleagues repeatedly go above and beyond what is expected of them for their patients. But we need help. We, and the children we care for, need governments to mend some of the existing fractures in holistic care for children – a group in society with no voice, no money and no vote.

Professor Sir Terence Stephenson DM, FRCPCH, FRCP
Nuffield Professor of Child Health, Institute of Child Health, UCL

Note

1 *Health and social care integration*. Department of Health, Department for Communities and Local Government and NHS England. HC 1011 SESSION 2016-17, 8 February 2017.

PREFACE

In August 1973 a public enquiry began in Brighton into the death of Maria Colwell. She was seven when she died of multiple injuries, sustained over a period of time, at the hands of her stepfather, William Kepple. Before her death Maria had been known to her school teachers, the newly formed East Sussex social services department, her GP, the NSPCC and other professionals. However, worried reports from neighbours to the NSPCC and the engagement of a range of statutory agencies did not prevent Maria's sad life and death (1). In the last nine months of Maria's life there had been 30 concerns raised about her welfare, by a number of people.

The death of a child under such circumstances is itself cause for a public outcry, but was increased by events that had taken place two years earlier. In 1971, and following a report chaired by Lord Frederic Seebohm, local authority social services departments had been established to bring together a range of previously separate agencies. In the words of what became known as the Seebohm report "a new department to meet the social needs of individuals, families and communities, which would incorporate the present functions of children's and welfare departments" (2, p. 43) would, for the first time, combine the work of Children's Departments, welfare services, education welfare and child guidance, mental health social work services and the social work services provided by health departments.

One of the major cases for change, which led to the Seebohm report, was the perennial problem of poor coordination between these organisations. Now there was the real possibility of a seamless service. The enquiry was determined, in its own words, to consider the personal social services in the broadest possible way, looking not only at the work of Children's Departments and welfare departments but the social work elements in health, education and housing. Yet, two years later, this new and brave new world of generic social services departments was perceived to be failing, allowing children to fall through a newly constructed safety net just established for their protection.

The challenge of uncoordinated services is one of the themes that runs throughout this book, like the place name in a stick of rock. It will be argued that whether services are run by health, education, social care, youth services or leisure, housing, the voluntary and private sector or the police there has been a lack of "joined up", "holistic" or "wraparound" care that is more frequently honoured in the breach than the observance.

Yet this is not the only theme the book will explore. In order to understand what is happening to children's services today, whoever the provider might be, it is first necessary to grasp how these structures have evolved. And, in this respect, what makes the book unusual, is that it traces these across health, social care and education, for example, rather than follow the trajectory of a single agency. So, in arriving at our present position it is, for example, necessary to understand the consequences of the Boer War on the nation's health; the seismic changes that accompanied the Second World War and that led to the establishment of the NHS, the 1944 Education Act, the raising of the school leaving age and the 1948 National Assistance Act, the establishment of academy schools and the 2012 Health and Social Care Act; all of which have fundamentally changed how we care for children.

These defining changes have, however, been accompanied by a gamut of post-Second World War initiatives, across all children's sectors, which in their, sometimes, brief incarnations have aimed to improve services for young people and, in common with one of the book's themes, were targeted at the greater integration of services.

If the argument is to be sustained that we can do much better to improve the lives of children, then objective evidence is needed both to demonstrate how we are failing and how well or not we perform against other European countries. Against a range of indicators, examining, for example, health, education or poverty, the UK's performance can be looked at against comparable countries and conclusions drawn.

Alongside a statistical analysis, we will also be looking at the economics of caring for children. How much does it all cost to care for children and how are the budgets divided? It is customary in most contemporary analyses of social policy to conclude with a plea for more resources and bigger budgets to meet rising demand. But the overall budget, dedicated to children's services and across all agencies, can stand the scrutiny of a more nuanced examination, where, it is argued, it might just be more a question of redistribution than the requirement to provide extra funding. This is particularly the case in relation to some of the short-term government initiatives, referred to earlier, and explored in greater detail later in the book.

The book will return to the theme of integration, providing examples, again both from the UK and other European countries, as to how bringing various agencies together, often on a small scale, has worked or where it has been very much needed but is not much in evidence. Comparisons can be made here with services for elderly people, where the imperative to bring health and social care together, for example, is driven by the need to release hospital beds by finding accommodation back in the community for discharged patients.

If this book is to have any impact, it clearly has to be about coming up with solutions and not just a restatement of the problems. And so a model for the integration of services is proposed. For the reader who has followed the book's journey so far, there will doubtless be a passionate belief that we could and should do more and better for children. My own career has corresponded with the journey from Seebohm to the separation of children and adult services, the widespread commissioning of health services, the privatisations of some children's services and a model of education that looks very different from the only distinction, being largely a binary one between grammar and secondary modern schools. It has led to a growing personal conviction that we owe children much more and could do things much better. The 2007 UNICEF statement has stood the test of time in asserting that:

> the true measure of a nation's standing is how well it attends to its children-their health and safety, their material security, their education and socialization and their sense of being loved, valued and included in the families and societies into which they are born.
>
> *(3, p. 3)*

Nothing else matters as much.

Notes

1 *Report of the Committee of Inquiry into the care and supervision provided in relation to Maria Colwell.* Department of Health and Social Security, 1974, HMSO, London.
2 *Report of the Committee on Local Authority and Allied Personal Social Services.* Home Department, the Secretary of State for Education and Science, the Minister of Housing and Local Government, and the Minister of Health 1968, HMSO, Cmnd 3703, London.
3 *Child poverty in perspective: an overview of child wellbeing in rich countries.* UNICEF, 2007, Innocenti Research Centre, Florence.

1

INTRODUCTION

Contemporary childhood

It is the best of times; it is the worst of times. It is the age of limitless information; it is the age of borderless social media. It is the epoch of wide opportunity; it is the era of unprecedented competition. It is a century of healthier, better educated children; it is a time of disturbing sexual abuse. We have all before us and yet we inhabit a hothouse of growing social pressures. Of no age group are these factors more true than that of the young growing up both in the UK and in other European countries today.

For contemporary children and young people, one of the newest and biggest challenges is that of choice. Thirty years ago, for example, about 14% of 18–21-year-olds attended university. Today, it is closer to 30%. Between 2016 and 2017 there were 2.32 million students studying at over 160 UK higher education institutions (excluding further education colleges) in a previously unforeseen range of vocational and non-vocational subjects. Two litmus tests for the way in which higher education has been extended to a wider cross section of young people is, first, that in 2016 English pupils receiving free school meals were 78% more likely to go to university than they were as little as ten years ago. Between 2008 and 2009, 17% of state-funded pupils who received free school meals entered higher education at 19. By 2014/15 this had risen to 24%. Second, that the number of full-time undergraduates from black and minority ethnic groups rose by 38% between 2007/8 and 2015/16 (1).

Children and young people are the most likely to be what Mark Prensky defined in 2001 as "digital natives", comfortable with new technology and quick to grasp the significance, amongst other things, of quicker, faster ways of doing things electronically. (We will later consider the downside of this.) Similarly, with advances in medicine and more attention to child safety than in the past, children's well-being is largely better than it has ever been. Fewer children die in the UK than they did

50 years ago and the major cause of child morbidity is no longer infectious disease (2). It is also the case that, as a result of Article 12 of the 1989 United Nations Convention on the Rights of the Child – the right to be heard – young people have a stronger voice and more say in some of the decisions that affect them.

What is not always understood is that the concept of childhood – particularly in literature – is a relatively recent idea. Peter Coveney traced it back to the end of the eighteenth century when, with writers like Wordsworth and Blake, the "romantic child" with sensibilities and a unique series of views on the world was first accepted (3). Similarly, Helen Seaford argued that early fifteenth- and sixteenth-century pictures show children as mini adults, dressed in heavy, ornate costumes. It is not until the nineteenth century that they are seen differently. High levels of infant mortality meant that it was not possible to take a sentimental view of children (4).

Now childhood and children with their own legal rights and voices is firmly established in the UK, although often couched in two contradictory sets of arguments. On the one hand is a view that the period of childhood, as such, is becoming shorter; the result of earlier physical maturity and increased pressure to grow up. This is largely encouraged by social media and commercial organisations keen to take a share of young people's growing economic power. On the other hand there is a move to heighten the age limit for children who are receiving some statutory services. The Chief Medical Officer's 2013 report on children's health used 25 as the cut-off date for some children's services. The justification being, first, that many adult services don't begin at 16 or 18 but sometimes much later than this (5). Second, that key elements of development, particularly emotional development, continue until the early 20s.

Despite the greater emphasis on children's rights, campaigning organisations point out that there remain wide anomalies in legal triggers to achieve adulthood. So, for example, you can marry at 16, with parental consent: the same age at which you can join the armed forces. You only need to be 14 before you can get a firearms licence, 17 before you can usually drive a car and 18 before you can buy alcohol in a pub or off-licence. There is no single law that defines the age of a child across the UK. The UN Convention on the Rights of the Child ratified by the UK in 1991 states that a child "means every human being below the age of eighteen years unless, under the law applicable to the child, majority is attained earlier" (6, p. 4). In the UK specific age limits are set out in relevant laws or government guidance. There are, however, differences between the UK nations. In England, Working Together 2013 refers to children up to their 18th birthday. In Wales, for example, the *All Wales Child Protection Procedures* states "A child is anyone who has not reached their 18th birthday". Children, therefore, means "children and young people" throughout (7, p. 17). The fact that a child has become 16 years of age, is living independently, is in further education, is a member of the armed forces, is in prison or a young offenders' institution does not change their status or their entitlement to services or protection under the Children Act 1989. For the purpose of this book, therefore, children are defined as all of those children and young people who have not yet reached their 18th birthday.

The pyramid of need

Given that the main focus of this book rests on what happens to those children – and their childhoods – when services fail, it is important to begin with the assertions of success, outlined above that many children navigate a successful route between the Scylla of state health, education, recreation or social welfare services and the Charybdis of pressure from social media and the demands of twenty-first-century life. They, however, are not the book's concern. Instead, the emphasis here is on those in need, from a variety of causes, and where the State has a duty to provide additional layers of support.

There have been numerous classifications of need, aiming either at a generic classification or that of a specific profession. It is best characterised by a simple pyramid, which is then subdivided in a range of slightly differing ways. Basic divisions are between intensive help, medium support and signposting to agencies offering some additional help. According to which model is being used, it is usually the level of "medium" support that tends to be the subject of further subdivision. So, if we provide two examples, children with significant health needs and those with mental health issues, we find that both often have a fourfold classification. A typical mental health model might begin with a simple referral through primary care, such as to a health visitor – tier 1. Tier 2 is to a specific mental health worker in primary care, say for counselling. Tier 3 relates to referrals to specialist child and adolescent workers and tier 4 referrals for specialist day or in-patient unit support. In the case of children with significant health issues, the tiers will move from support provided within primary care to Level 4 where intervention may be at the level of palliative care or for children with life-threatening conditions.

The book proposes a four-tier pyramid, where help gradually becomes more intensive. If we look at the normal distribution of children and young people across a typical population, we find that the level of need falls crudely into this four-tier pyramid. At the base of the pyramid are the majority of young people, capable of growing by accessing main stream services, such as education or health. Above, at tier 2, there is a cohort where some degree of support is necessary. They may, for example, require additional educational help because of dyslexia, speech or language difficulties or parenting programmes requiring some additional help, if only to prevent problems from escalating.

At tier 3 are those who will need some specialist services and staff. This may be because of a disability, school exclusion, issues of homelessness or because of already experienced mental health problems. At the top, tier 4, are children and young people with high dependency needs. This may be a life-threatening condition, the requirement to provide palliative care, complex educational needs or, for example, because they are looked-after children in the care of the local authority. The book's focus is on tiers 3 and 4 and this model assumes that the high costs of intervention will lie in tiers 3 and 4. The relationship between individual assessments – by a specific profession – and the devising of an overall, generic and multi-disciplinary score will be explored in Chapter 8.

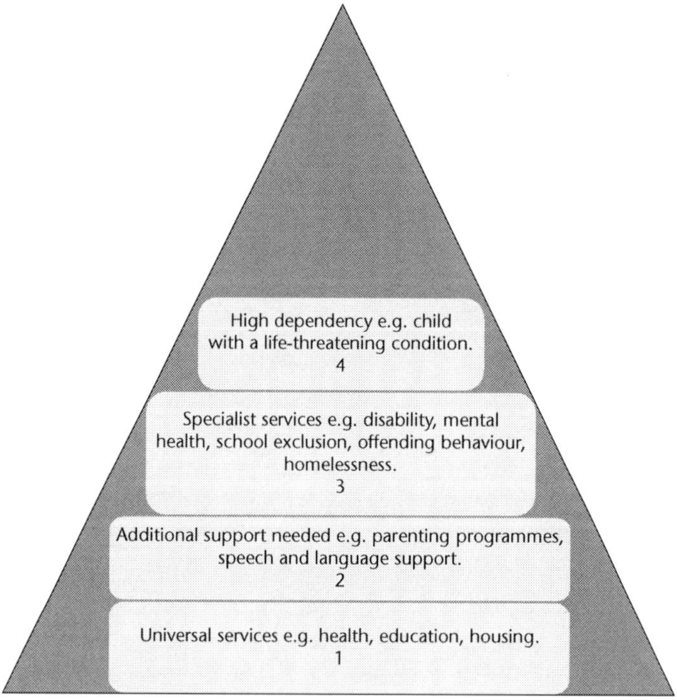

FIGURE 1.1 Pyramid of need

The protection of children

What the remainder of Chapter 1 explores is, albeit selectively, examples of failure and disconnected services from a wide range of statutory and voluntary agencies. It is an examination of what has gone wrong, in order to extract some over-arching lessons, which need addressing if services are to improve. Often, they concern children already identified as both vulnerable and requiring special help – the top tier 4 of the pyramid. The way they have been widely reported is equally important, as this helps to illustrate a central argument about the fragmentation of current services. Taking as examples the Rotherham child sexual exploitation inquiry, the deaths of Daniel Pelka, Kaiya Blake, Ben, Max and Olivia Clarence, the exclusion of very young children from schools, the 2010 Kennedy Inquiry into NHS services for children and the Children Commissioner's 2018 Vulnerability Report, all help to illustrate not only that we face major challenges across a wide range of agencies, including health, education and social care, but that these are often exacerbated by a systemic failure of what we will come to see as non- integrated services.

The *Independent Inquiry into Child Sexual Exploitation in Rotherham* published in 2014 (8) revealed that between 1997 and 2013 over 1,400 children had been sexually abused by groups of mostly Asian men. The true scale of abuse is not known but included rape by multiple perpetrators, and girls trafficked to other towns and cities in the north of England, abducted, beaten and intimidated. Just over a third of those affected were previously known to services, because of issues surrounding child protection and neglect. Tangentially, this finding is confirmed by other studies that have examined the large number of children and young people in care who go missing every year. In a report recorded by Young Minds, the NSPCC estimated that in 2012, for example, more than 3,000 children went missing from care on 28,000 occasions (9).

Evidence from the subsequent Rotherham inquiry, chaired by Alexis Jay, indicated that despite the warnings of youth workers, the police in Yorkshire gave no priority to child sexual exploitation and the actions of social services to respond to the abuse allegations were largely too little and too late. There was similarly no engagement with leaders of the Pakistani heritage community, to discuss how they could best jointly address the issues. In a series of recommendations, Professor Jay stated that the authority should develop a more strategic approach to sexually exploited children and there should be much closer working arrangements between a whole range of agencies.

Subsequently, further and similar investigations for comparable alleged crimes were conducted by police forces across the country, with groups of men prosecuted for the organised sexual grooming of victims, in areas as distant and different as Oxford, Leeds, High Wycombe, Halifax and Newcastle. While wider factors have come into play, influencing the way these crimes have been understood and reported, there has been a failure to listen to the voices of young people, coupled with separate services all failing to act in a concerted way. A factor we will explore in other areas of the care of children.

Rotherham was largely the result of a collective failure by the police and social services. In the case of children Ben, Max and Olivia Clarence, the *dramatis personae* was much wider. In 2014 Tania Clarence, the mother of the three children, was sentenced after a verdict of manslaughter against all the children, on the grounds of diminished responsibility. All three children had spinal muscular atrophy and had received services from a range of statutory agencies. The subsequent serious case review (10) revealed that there had been over 80 health professionals, GPs and social workers involved with the family. This included a designated nurse, nine health organisations, the local authority children's social care departments, two schools and a spinal muscular atrophy charity. Gary Clarence, Tania's husband, stated that the range of differing professionals, all making decisions about what was in the best interest of the children, meant that as a couple they were always trying to balance their medical needs with the desire to provide the children with as warm and as normal a life as possible. The Serious Case Review argued that it was not always clear whom the lead professional was and noted that, at one stage, the family had asked for an intermediary to help deal with the sheer number of staff and agencies assigned to work with them. Part of this evidence recalls services before the Seebohm report, described earlier, where families could receive help from a myriad of professional workers.

In a subsequent *Sunday Times* investigation (11), a similar situation is quoted in which "Ben", also diagnosed with spinal muscular atrophy, had 271 appointments, with more than 60 professionals in 50 different departments and in 17 different locations. Clearly, the complexity of these children's needs demands a response from a wide range of agencies, although arguments as to whether we are delivering services in the best way remain to be answered. This example seems a long way from the American concept of "wraparound care", where a child's needs are dealt with comprehensively by a small group of professionals working collectively and to which we will return in Chapter 7.

Similar questions surround the death of Daniel Pelka, who at the age of four was murdered by his mother and her partner. Daniel died in 2012 and for several months before his death had been both starved and beaten. At his death he was grossly malnourished, dehydrated and had bruises all over his body. The *Serious Case Review*, published the following year (12) reveals that Daniel had been known to doctors, teachers and teaching assistants, social care and the police. Indeed, the police had been called to his carers' home on 26 separate occasions, as a result of domestic abuse. Despite Daniel scavenging food from school rubbish bins and eating beans from gardening trays, while the class was planting them, there was a failure by the agencies to coordinate the information that might have saved his life. The serious case review identified concerns relating to information sharing and communication between professions: namely teachers, social workers, health professionals and the police. No one had a complete picture of Daniel's life. It is worth recalling Daniel's tragic circumstances in mind, when we come to look at the Multi-Agency Safeguarding Hubs examined in Chapter 7.

Young people and mental health

Echoing this view – about the need for coordinated services – was the inquiry *Getting It Right for Children and Young People*, undertaken by Sir Ian Kennedy in 2010 (13). Ten years earlier Kennedy had investigated serious failings in cardiac surgery in Bristol, where children had died or were seriously damaged by the treatment they received. There had been a number of tragic and high profile cases since the 2001 report on Bristol Royal Infirmary, including, for example, the death of Peter Connelly in 2007. He concluded that, more generally, nationwide care for children was subordinated to the demands of adults. For example, only 12% of the health budget was spent on children. The 2010 report presented an opportunity to revisit some of these issues, to reflect the frustration often expressed by parents and carers at the lack of coordination between services. Kennedy explored the complex array and interplay of organisations, units and teams and highlighted the NHS's lack of "join up" with other services. This, he argued, was often a frustration to parents and carers where, for example (and, as we saw in the case of the Clarence family), appointments are scheduled on consecutive days and at multiple locations when arranging them in the same place on the same day would save a long journey and time off work. Kennedy also pointed to the isolation of policy for children and young people's health and welfare, separate from those wider policies for children. This has two effects, forcing care for children and young people into an unwinnable battle with adult care and frustrating local cooperation as differences in departments' philosophies are played out in practice.

Lastly, Kennedy points specifically at GP training, noting that GPs often have little or no experience of paediatrics as part of their professional training. Altogether, he concludes:

> the ultimate goal must be to shift the focus away from single professional units and identities, with their particular goals, to a single minded concern only for the outcomes that are needed for children and young people: that is, work backwards and start with the child or young person ("I exist to provide for you"), rather than forwards from "This is what I, as a professional do".
>
> *(13, p. 14)*

Kennedy's comments, although aimed specifically at the better coordination of health services, have a wider applicability to other care organisations. In September 2011, Kaiya Blake, aged four, was suffocated by her mother, Chantelle, who was diagnosed with delusions, hallucinations and paranoid schizophrenia. The Serious Case Review in 2013 by Manchester's Safeguarding Board (14) indicated that there had been previous involvement from Manchester Children's Social Care, Manchester Early Years and Sure Start, the Greater Manchester Police, Addactus Housing, NHS Manchester, Manchester Mental Health and Social Care Trust and the Central Manchester Foundation Trust. Like Maria Colwell, in 1973 there had been reports from the public of violence seen by others towards Kaiya. Furthermore, the approach to case planning had been "fairly chaotic" and the review concluded that much of the emphasis from workers had been on Chantelle's mental illness and not on Kaiya.

Individual examples of inadequate mental health services – as evidenced by Tania Clarence and Kaiya's mother – point to more major failings in mental health for children and young people. Three major challenges to existing services have emerged with some degree of regularity – local investment in Child and Adolescent Mental Health Services (CAMHS), the availability of beds for those requiring in-patient treatment and transition services for those moving from adolescent to adult care. Despite recent assertions about the need for "parity of esteem" between mental and physical health, there is evidence that mental health remains very much the poor relation.

A lot of mental illness has its origins in the teenage years, which is why the establishment of CAMHS teams was seen as both a preventive and reactive response to young people experiencing difficulties with their emotional and behavioural well-being. The development of CAMHS began in 1998 with a four tier pyramid or system ranging from general advice and treatment for less severe problems to highly specialist services for children and young people with serious mental health issues. The spectrum of support offered by CAMHS embraces depression, anorexia and other, largely adolescent, eating disorders, self-harm and violence, to schizophrenia. CAMHS teams include psychiatrists, psychologists, social workers, nursing staff and occupational therapists but receiving support is sometimes difficult and can depend on where you live. A review of CAMHS in 2008 not only revealed wide regional variations in services but the need for "organisations and professions to work effectively together around children and families" (15). Then, following a 2014 parliamentary Health and Select Committee investigation, a review promised increased funding for mental health services. Unfortunately, not all of this has been released. A report by the National Health Executive, in 2016, revealed that only about 0.7% of the total NHS budget was allocated to children's mental health services and even when extra money was allocated, unless specifically "ring-fenced" it was used to support other services (16). While help may vary – depending upon where in the country you live – the concept of providing support for young people with mental health problems through a range of professionals is one to which we will return.

For those requiring some form of in-patient mental health treatment the paucity of help has been widely reported. Accounts of young people having to travel hundreds of miles to receive treatment are usually accompanied by details of how this has affected family life. Figures from the Mental Welfare Commission for Scotland, for example, reveal that in 2016 of the 17 patients in the Priory Eating Disorder Unit in Glasgow, 13 were from England. The Commission revealed that 90% of patients being treated at two specialist eating disorder clinics in Scotland had been sent hundreds of miles from their home in England, by the NHS. Seven separate health authorities, from as far afield as Kent and Buckinghamshire, had sent patients to the private Priory Hospital in Glasgow (17).

Lastly, in relation to child mental health services, is the issue of making the transition to adult services. This move from CAMHS to Adult Mental Health services should take place at 18, but a report for the Joint Commissioning Panel for Mental Health, from the Royal College of Psychiatrists pointed to the disconnect between the two services. Up to a third of teenagers are lost somewhere between children's and adult services and a further third experienced an interruption in their care (18). When this is exacerbated by young people having to travel hundreds of miles before a bed can be found, for inpatient treatment, the problems are particularly acute.

Youth justice

There are interesting parallels to be drawn between the difficulties experienced by mental health services for children and young people and what has happened to youth justice services in the UK. The Youth Justice Board, which has overall responsibility for young offender services, came into being after the 1998 Crime and Disorder Act of the same year – with the aim of preventing the offending and re-offending of young people. The Youth Offending services work with young people between the ages of 10 and 17 and consist of three major components – Youth Offending Teams (YOTs), introduced in Section 39 of the Crime and Disorder Act, community youth justice services and what is known as the youth secure estate. Youth Offending Teams are, like CAMHS services, delivered locally with social services and education and in partnership with the police, probation and health authorities. For those requiring support and containment the Youth Justice Board contracts with providers for secure children's homes, secure training centres and young offender institutions. The overall budget on the Youth Justice Board has been cut between 2015 and 2017, with expenditure of £210.2 million in 2016/17, representing a reduction of £18m or 7.9% compared to 2015/16 (19). These cuts, it is argued, can lead to a greater use of residential secure accommodation, if community support is not available.

The concept of locally managed, community services aiming to prevent young people needing residential or secure accommodation and provided by a range of professionals is very similar to the thinking behind CAMHS. When functioning well, YOTs work alongside the police, health and housing services, concentrating, wherever possible on prevention. For those who require some form of secure accommodation, there is a correlation between previous periods in care and earlier abuse or neglect at home. A 2012 report, from the Howard League for Penal Reform, revealed that 71% of children in custody had been involved with or had been in the care of the social services, compared with 3% of the general population. One in four boys reported suffering violence at home and one in twenty had been sexually abused. In total, 31% had a recognised mental health disorder (compared with 10% of the general population) and 86% of boys and 82% of girls had been excluded from school (20). The theme of early intervention, like that of multi-disciplinary and integrated working is, again, one which the book will explore in further detail.

Coupled with pressure on youth justice budgets has been a gradual reduction in what are described as non-statutory youth services. A Unison report in 2016 stated that in the two financial years 2014/15 and 2015/16 cuts in youth services amounted to £123 million (21). Between 2014 and 2016, 244 youth centres were closed, youth clubs ceased and, again, the preventive work aimed at keeping young people out of the juvenile justice system became more of a challenge. Almost 98,000 youth service places for young people were cut between 2014 and 2016. Evidence also indicates that this failure to invest in some services for children, such as youth clubs, which can be seen as having an important preventive role, has also extended to other non-statutory services. In 2014, following a Freedom of Information request, *Children and Young People Now* (22), revealed that one in three local authorities had closed some staffed and unstaffed play provision since 2011. These have mostly been the result of a 38% fall in councils' overall spending on play between 2010 and 2013. Responses from 157 councils responsible for play in England – a combination of county, borough, city, town and district councils – revealed that on average 2.4% of an area's total play provision had been lost. While cutting outdoor play space could be seen as an easy target for stretched local authorities, as we shall subsequently argue, the ability to play outdoors should be an essential ingredient of every child's life.

At the same time, increased diversity and complexity in the way that education is provided to children and young people has resulted in both greater challenges for integration of services and rising trends in school exclusion – as a litmus test that education is failing some pupils. Between 2015 and 2016, there were 6,685 permanent exclusions – a rise of 27% on the previous year's figure of 5,785 (23). Rates of expulsions at primary and secondary schools in England have risen every year since 2012/13. Of equal concern are the number of expulsions – some of children as young as five, for sexual misconduct, including abuse, assault, and harassment and watching pornography. Figures obtained via a Freedom of Information request by the Press Association from 15 local authorities found 754 children either expelled or temporarily excluded from school as a result of sexual misconduct in the last four years. At least 40 cases involved children under 10 (24).

Lastly, in relation to those young people who are at the top of any pyramid of need, is the second report from the English Children's Commissioner on vulnerable young people (25). It moves on from quantifying the level of childhood vulnerability in England, recorded in a previous report, to more about the children themselves growing up with risks. The report concludes that 2.1 million children in England (1 in 6) are living vulnerable lives, due to complex family circumstances. Of these 1.6m are receiving no known support or help from the system. Furthermore:

- 825,000 children are living in a family with domestic violence and over 100,000 children are living in a family with what the report describes as the "toxic trio" of domestic violence, mental health and alcohol or substance abuse;
- 890,000 children live with parents suffering serious mental health problems;
- 825,000 children live in households with domestic violence;
- 470,000 children live with parents who use substances "problematically";
- 170,000 children care for their parents or siblings.

And as the report points out, because they don't receive early intervention, they can go on to put huge pressures on family courts, schools and the care system.

Establishing what is really happening to children

The argument was made, at the outset of this chapter, that many children emerge from childhood not only unscathed but better educated than their parents; much healthier than children a generation ago and ready for their lives to be filled with opportunities scarcely dreamt of, even 20 years ago. Within this context, the above examples of cuts to services, failures to protect vulnerable children and examples of variable care across the UK could be seen as playing into the hands of the popular press, keen to expose a wide spectrum of children's scandals. And establishing well researched truth into what is *really* happening to children is tricky – particularly in relation to those vulnerable children at the apex of the pyramid. For some areas of care for children we haven't been collecting statistics long enough to make valid comparisons between years; some challenges such as Internet abuse remain new and in some cases public attitudes to, say, child abuse offences, have changed.

Colin Pritchard, for example, who has researched widely in the field of child abuse, argues that the popular emphasis on failure masks the wider successes of many services. However, "demonstrating successful prevention is impossible, as it is trying to prove a negative" (26). UK figures, for example, look particularly favourable when compared with the USA.

Contrary to this is the 2017 Ofsted report looking at serious incident notifications involving death or serious harm to a child when abuse or neglect is known or suspected. Between 2016 and 2017 there were 433 serious incident notifications; this was a 14% increase on the number of notifications in 2015/16. Also, the number of deaths has gone up in the same period. There were 211 cases of child death, compared with 171 in the previous year and 163 between 2013 and 2014 (27). UK figures, for example, look particularly favourable, he argued, when compared with the USA.

Another attempt at demonstrating whether the figures for child protection are improving or declining is provided by a 2017 report from the NSPCC. It looked at child protection from the perspective of 20 indicators, including child homicides, the number of recorded sexual offences and also recorded cruelty or neglect, and violent incidents experienced by 10–15-year-olds (28). The report concludes that since 2009 there has been a 39% increase in children on child protection plans, an 80% increase in calls to the NSPCC helpline, a 109% increase in police recorded sexual offences and a 298% increase in police recorded indecent image offences. But, as the report cautions, this could reflect an increased awareness by people generally of child protection issues as much as a greater number of children being abused.

We can confidently assert, however, that it is an impossibility child abuse could ever be fully eradicated. But with accurate records only going back over a relatively short period of time, we need to be circumspect about any conclusions we draw.

But enough evidence has been provided to begin to draw some conclusions on contemporary services for children in the UK. First, failure to protect children is not the fault of a single discipline, but can be seen across health, social care, education, the police and the voluntary sector. Second, that failure is often the result of a lack of integration – of agencies just not working together and thereby creating gaps through which children fall. Third, that some cuts to what might be regarded as preventive services can serve to put young people on a path to more intrusive and often more far reaching (sometimes) residential intervention. So, the failure of a local CAMH's service, supporting a young person with mental health problems in the community, might lead, eventually, to in-patient treatment, just as a reduction in youth facilities leads to custodial options. This is clearly never simply a matter of cause and effect, but some links are there.

While this chapter has served to show where some of the current challenges are, it is now important both to demonstrate how these services have evolved and also how care for children in the UK compares with that of other European countries. The book will then examine a wide range of government initiatives, following the Second World War – most of which have attempted to address some of the shortfalls analysed above. From this position we can explore what full integration might mean to the lives of vulnerable young people.

Notes

1 *Widening participation in higher education, England. 2014–15 age cohort.* August 2017, Department of Education, London.
2 *Growing up in the UK. Ensuring a health future for our children.* BMA, 2013, Board of Science, London.
3 *The image of childhood.* Coveney, P., 1967, Peregrine Books, London. First published as *Poor Monkey*, 1957, Rockliff.
4 Children and childhood: perceptions and realities. Seaford, H., 2001, *The Political Quarterly*, vol 72, issue 4.
5 *Chief Medical Officer annual report 2012: children and young people's health.* Davies, S., 2013, Department of Health and Social Security.
6 *UN convention on the rights of the child 1989, article 1.* Office of the High Commissioner for Human Rights, Article 1, 1989.
7 *All Wales child protection procedures – children in Wales 2008.* Produced on behalf of all Local Safeguarding Children's Boards in Wales
8 *Independent inquiry into child exploitation in Rotherham 1997–2013.* Jay, A., 2014, Rotherham Metropolitan Borough Council, Rotherham.
9 Reported in *Young Minds*, Summer 2013, issue 120.
10 *Family a serious case review findings.* London Borough of Kingston upon Thames Local Safeguarding Children's Board, 2015.
11 It's so hard for me to take her life. Driscoll, M., *Sunday Times*, 23 November 2014.
12 *Serious case review. Re: Daniel Pelka 2007–2012.* Coventry Local Safeguarding Board, 2013, Coventry.
13 *Getting it right for children and young people. Overcoming cultural barriers in the NHS so as to meet their needs.* Kennedy, Sir Ian, September 2010, Department of Health and Social Care, Kingston Upon Thames.
14 *Serious case review in relation to Kaiya Blake*, Manchester Safeguarding Children's Board, 2013, Manchester.
15 *Children and young people in mind. The final report of the national CAMHS review.* Chair, Davidson, Jo 2008, Department for Children, Schools and Families and the Department of Health, London.
16 *CAMHS cash at risk of being diverted from frontline.* Mental Health National Health Executive, 2016, London, press release.
17 *Report on unannounced visit to the Priory Hospital.* Mental Welfare Commission for Scotland, 2017, Mental Welfare Commission for Scotland, Edinburgh.
18 *Mental health services for young people making the transition from child and adolescent to adult services.* Royal Commissioning Panel for Mental Health, 2012, Practical Mental Health Commissioning, vol 2.
19 *Annual report and accounts 2016–17.* The Youth Justice Board for England and Wales, 2017, Youth Justice Board, London.
20 *Future insecure. Secure children's homes in England and Wales.* The Howard League for Penal Reform, 2012, The Howard League for Penal Reform, London.
21 *The damage. A future at risk. Cuts in youth services.* Unison, 2016, Unison, London.
22 Outdoor play under threat from local facilities and funding cull. Jozwiak, G., 7 January 2014, *Children and Young People Now.*
23 *Permanent and fixed period exclusions 2015 to 2016.* Department for Education, 20 July 2017, Department for Education, Darlington.

24 Schools exclude five year olds for sexual misconduct. Weale, S., 9 August 2017, *The Guardian*.
25 *Vulnerability report 2018, overview*. Children's Commissioner, 2018, Children's Commissioner for England, London.
26 Violent death of children in England and Wales and the major possible evidence of improving child protection. Pritchard, C. and Williams, R., 2010, *Child Abuse Review*, vol 17, issue 5, pp. 289–364.
27 *Serious incident notification from local authority children's services 2016 to 2017: main findings*. Ofsted, 2017, Ofsted.
28 *How safe are our children? The most comprehensive overview of child protection in the UK*. Bentley, H., O'Hagan, O., Brown, A., Vasco, N., Lynch, C., Peppiate, J., Webber, M., Ball, R., Miller, P., Byrne, A., Hofizi, M. and Letendrie, F., 2017, NSPCC.

2

"THE FIVE GIANT EVILS"

An historical perspective on services for children

The Boer War

Out of a cohort of 11,000 male Manchester volunteers, 8,000 were rejected. In order to fight in the infantry and take part in the 1899–1902 Boer War, men needed to be five foot three inches tall, to have a chest measurement of at least 33 inches and to weigh at least 8 stone 3 pounds (1). Instead, most men were turned down as short-sighted, pigeon-chested, suffering from fallen arches, rickets, diminutive, diseased or otherwise "substandard" (2). That Britain struggled to crush a tiny nation of isolated Afrikaners, begged the inevitable question as to what would happen with a more powerful enemy and triggered a debate about "national efficiency" and, in particular, the physical condition of the urban working class. There was a perceived bond between physical deficiency, intellectual inefficiency and inadequate nutrition and, as the historian Bentley Gilbert's caustic view had it, there was an influential belief that "an unhealthy schoolchild was a danger to all society and, that it was in society's selfish, non- humanitarian interest to see that the child was (medically) treated" (3, p. 14). Hence, a scare over what appeared to be a deterioration in fitness led to serious political questions being asked. As Lloyd George summarised the national mood, Britain could not run an "A1" empire equipped with a "C3" population.

These events corresponded with reports into poverty by social reformers, such as Charles Booth's first scientific estimates of poverty and investigations into its causes and Seebohm Rowntree's parallel work on both poverty and nutrition. They calculated that up to 30% of the population of the cities were living in or below poverty levels and were often caught up in situations from which they could not extricate themselves. These reports were also in parallel with the needs of a new Liberal government to have a strong social programme that would compete with the growing power of the Labour party. While the Labour Party were campaigning for social welfare policies, such as old age and unemployment benefits, the Liberals were turning away from a laissez-faire approach to social reform, towards a programme of positive action. After all, and in relation to children, and mirroring earlier comments, "an unhealthy schoolchild was a danger to all society" (3, p. 14). The result was a wealth of legislation, which, depending upon your viewpoint, aimed at an overall improvement in the general welfare of British children or cannon fodder for the next war.

Two government inquiries were crucial. The 1903 Report of the Royal Commission on Physical Training stated that physical welfare of the population was seriously impacted by lack of proper nourishment. In the following year an inter-departmental committee on Physical Deterioration concluded that the "evils" arising from underfeeding were widespread and in need of urgent attention (3). It led both to the passing of the Education (Provision of Meals) Act, 1906, and the Education (Administrative Provisions) Act the following year.

The first of these, the Education (Provision of Meals) Act, 1906, gave local education authorities powers to "take such steps as they think fit for the provision of meals for children in attendance at any public elementary school in their area". It followed on from schemes, in the 1880s, usually run by voluntary agencies, as far apart as Edinburgh, Glasgow, Manchester and London to provide usually hot meals, once or twice a week for poor families. There had been a widespread debate as to whether these should be free or the voluntary agencies should be enabled to charge a small free. The argument for the charge was that free meals would "pauperise" families whom, instead, should be assisted to maintain themselves and carry out their parental responsibilities (3).

The Education (Administrative Provisions) Act, 1907 created a duty on local education authorities to "provide for the medical inspection of children immediately before or at the time of or as soon as possible after their admission to a public elementary school" (3, p. 114). In practice, it was intended that the School Medical Officer would carry out a number of different functions, examining all children on entry into school, combat common diseases and physical unfitness and check that school rooms were properly ventilated and not over-crowded. By the conclusion of 1909 medical inspection schemes had been established in 307 out of 328 authorities (3).

These developments marked the first modern period where there was a significant and sustained attempt to improve the general welfare of children and young people. For the purposes of the book it is significant in two ways. First, because the social reforms were precipitated, by the nation standing back and finding itself wanting – as a result of the lessons of the Boer War. Second, because changes that resulted from this self-criticism outlasted the narrow confines of a single parliamentary cycle. The Liberal reforms remained in place after governments had changed and were built upon by subsequent reforming legislation. This becomes important when later (in Chapter 3) we will be considering the short-term nature of a lot of near contemporary government social reform initiatives for children, which rarely outlasted a single government.

The Second World War

To an even greater extent, these two criteria for significant change – crisis and sustainability – were evident in the social reform planning that took place during the Second World War. The extraordinary foresight that was shown in this period was the way in which, during the darkest days of the war, a vision emerged of what a new health, welfare and education system might look like. The overarching vision of the Labour government of 1945–51 under Clement Attlee was the provision of houses and jobs for all the servicemen and women returning from the war, the creation of free healthcare and a cradle-to-grave welfare system as a universal right, rather than subject to any means test. Slightly earlier, in 1942, the Beveridge Report had outlined proposals for destroying what were described at the "five giant evils" of "Want, Disease, Ignorance, Squalor and Idleness" (2). In 1942 what was eventually to become the NHS was being planned and co-incidentally Beveridge published his report on social insurance and allied services, three weeks after the Battle of Alamein, selling 100,000 copies in the first month.

It is almost impossible to over-emphasise the foresight of serious thinking about what a future world might look like, at a time when the very existence of that world must have seemed to be in doubt. Even the argument that it was important to have a vision to oppose the ideology of Nazi Germany does not seem sufficient to explain the prescience of those planning for a new post-war welfare state. And, ironically in this context, the Beveridge Report was not only translated into 22 languages and dropped over occupied Europe during the War, but copies were later discovered in German, in Hitler's bunker (2).

If the Boer War had seen some concerted, if limited, attempts to improve the lives of children, the period from 1944–48 resulted in a welter of legislation. Education reform was passed in the Butler Act of 1944, the Family Allowances Act, to provide child benefit, the following year and, in 1946 the Act to establish the NHS was passed. There had been consensus, pre-1939, that the existing system of National Health Insurance should be revised and the Second World War itself led to a new central emergency medical service for air raid victims. The scope of this service increased, as the war progressed, and in 1941 the government had pledged a national hospital service, after the war ended. The extent to which the NHS Act in 1946 went much further than emergency medical services was, again, a tribute to the creative thinking of these years. As Beveridge promised in the Beveridge Report 1942, "medical treatment covering all requirements will be provided for all citizens by a national health service" (n.p.). The National Insurance Act was approved in the same year and two years later, the National Assistance Act passed.

In a Fabian Society article Harrop concluded that:

> We should greet Beveridge at 70 as optimists. The Beveridge report is, after all, a reminder that it is possible to imagine and realise visionary yet practical reforms, even in times of crisis and severe financial constraint. The left

> should rightly celebrate how much of Beveridge's legacy lives on, especially in pensions and health. But we should also feel inspired by Beveridge's example to seek out comprehensive solutions to the giants we face today.
>
> *(4, p. 3)*

The National Assistance Act at last terminated the long established Poor Laws. Instead, it made provision for the welfare of disabled, sick, aged and other people and introduced the idea of a safety net for those who were not in a position to pay National Insurance contributions, such as homeless people. It established the National Assistance Board (to operate the National Assistance scheme) and, again, was passed in the spirit of honouring a financial commitment to many of those newly returned from the war. In another Fabian Society article, celebrating "Beveridge at 70", Byrne stated:

> Finally on the afternoon of 6 February 1946, the Minister of National Insurance, Jim Griffiths got to his feet to move the national insurance bill be read a second time. After years of preparation, a nation battered by war passed the Beveridge report into law. The lesson of history is clear; even in the toughest times our country can afford to put ambition into action when we act to put people into jobs.
>
> *(5, p. 14)*

While there have been considerable incremental changes to welfare benefits, since the passing of the 1948 National Assistance Act, the responsibility for its administration has largely remained a government responsibility. In 2012, for example, the Welfare Reform Act introduced the idea of Universal Credit, replacing six previously means tested benefits (including housing benefit, child tax benefit, income support and Jobseeker's Allowance). Many of the changes we shall later trace through health, social care and education, for example, have led to services being taken over by new providers, such as the private sector or voluntary organisations. In the case of welfare benefits this has not happened, but change has been driven by other fundamental differences to income support, which are the result of changes in political ideologies.

To a large extent all three political parties went to the election in 1945 committed to principles of social and economic reconstruction. Previously fought arguments about socialism, as opposed to a laissez-faire capitalism, were now replaced by pragmatic reform in a mixed economy (6). Also, the political consensus that had largely been retained together during the war, continued as all parties concentrated on getting Britain back on its feet.

The 1948 Children Act

Direct reform of social care services for children, during this period, came from a slightly different route. In the 1930s the Poor Law was criticised for the way it organised and ran residential homes for children. As a result, the functions were handed over to local authorities, who ran the homes through what were usually called Public Assistance Departments (7). The Second World War led to the evacuation of a large number of children and separation from their parents and carers. This, to some extent, helped to focus attention on children who, for a wide range of reasons, were living away from home. Marjory Allen, a child care pioneer, became at first interested and later deeply concerned at the drab and empty lives of those growing up in residential care. A letter to *The Times* from Marjory Allen about their plight, printed on 15 July 1944 brought to the attention of readers the state of children growing up in poor quality residential care:

> The social upheaval caused by the war has not only increased this army of unhappy children, but presents an opportunity for transforming their conditions. The Education Bill and the White Paper on the Health Services have alike ignored the problem and the opportunity.

The letter was followed by a pamphlet, the following year, entitled *Whose Children?* (8). This not only included accounts of the emptiness of the lives of many of the children in residential homes but pointed out that they were largely run by unqualified staff, who had been given little training. Lady Allen also identified that there were three Ministries responsible for these children (the Home Office, the Ministry of Health and the Ministry of Education) and argued that there was "considerable overlapping . . . in regard to the number of homes and the children therein".

This issue of split responsibility between government departments was one to which Lady Allen returned, in preparing evidence to the Curtis Committee, looking into the plight of children in the care system. In her private papers, held by the University of Warwick, she records:

> One of the most unfortunate features of the present system is that the overlapping of departmental functions has made it difficult to regard the child as an individual who needs continuity of method and environment.
>
> *(9)*

Here, again, is a theme to which we will frequently return.

1945 also saw the death of Denis O'Neill, a Welsh boy, at the hands of his foster parents, Mr and Mrs Gough. This led to an enquiry by Sir Walter Monkton and, in words that will already sound familiar to readers, the subsequent report indicated the absence of coordination between different authorities and showed that the problems of current child care were not confined to those in residential homes but to the way the whole system was administered. It led, via the Curtis Committee, mentioned above, and the 1946 Clyde Report on Homeless Children, chaired by James Clyde, to the passing of the 1948 Children Act and the establishment of new Children's Departments, which were then to remain in existence up to the passing of the Seebohm proposals discussed in the Preface.

The Children Act stipulated that local authorities take on the duty to receive children under the age of 17 into their care, when parents or carers were unable to provide for them and whose welfare required the intervention of the local authority. The Act established local authority children's committees, which were also to take over responsibility for children committed to local authorities by the courts, for the protection of private foster care, for the supervision of some adoption placements and for the inspection of voluntary homes. There was to be a new organisation – Children's Departments – ultimately under the control of the Home Office (7).

Aneurin Bevan's speech to the Executive Councils Association on 7 October 1948, that what was happening across health, national insurance, the care of children and their education "is the biggest single experiment in social services that the world has ever seen undertaken" is much more than the normal hype from zealous politicians. Like the social changes that were brought about by the Boer War, they were precipitated by crises and changes to the world order. They also saw through the vagaries of a single parliamentary cycle and were also brought about by a degree of party consensus. As the Liberals, after the Boer War, reached out to meet an emerging Labour Party agenda, so, too, the parties came together in the embers of the Second World War to embrace change values they all largely shared. This search for consensus and an over-arching vision to improve the lives of children, whether through education, a new NHS or reform of the national assistance system was the recipe for a way forward capable of creating permanent change. In Chapter 3, this will be contrasted with a range of more recent government initiatives, many of which were capable of effecting children's lives radically if they had been – like the establishment of the post-Second World War welfare state – both sustained and, as we shall also argue, properly evaluated.

The 1944 Education Act and the Seebohm Report

Finally, in the raft of Second World War legislation was the 1944 Education Act; no less radical than the other welfare reforms. R.A. Butler, ostensibly sidelined by Churchill into taking on the education portfolio in government, was quick to realise that it provided him with a unique opportunity to affect irretrievably the lives of children. Interestingly, Butler, a Conservative education secretary, worked in close cooperation with Labour's education expert James Chuter Ede, a teacher, trade unionist and Labour politician: another example of some of the welfare state consensus that steered the new welfare state.

The Act which was, in fact, passed during the war but only implemented when it had ended, made a clear delineation between primary (6–11 years old) and secondary (from 11 and then extended to 15) schools, with a tripartite system of grammar, secondary technical schools and secondary modern schools. It was followed by similar legislation in Scotland in 1945 (the Education (Scotland) Act) and also put a duty on local authorities to provide school meals and milk. It was described by one commentator at the time as a bill that gathers up the dreams of educational reformers and was a testament to Butler's political acumen. What he managed to do was appease the Conservatives (because it honoured religion and social hierarchy), pacify Labour (because it opened up new opportunities for working class children) and pleased the general public (because it ended the system of school fees). During its gestation it attracted a lot of interest and engagement from the public. My father's private diary of the time, usually solely preoccupied with how British troop movements were progressing across the world, recorded, on 24 October 1943, that "great interest is being shown in the new Education Bill". Its longevity was evidence of forward thinking where, again, the nation could have argued it was being distracted by world events.

Reference was made, in the book's Preface, to the 1968 Seebohm Report, which led to the establishment of new social services departments. Children's Departments, which had been established as a result of the 1948 Children Act, ceased to exist, subsumed into social services departments, which, it was argued, would be more capable of dealing holistically with a family's problems. No wonder, it might have been argued, that families never got on top of their social problems, if they had to deal with the relentless footfall of hospital almoners, welfare officers, mental welfare officers and probation officers crossing their front door! Now they would only need to provide tea and biscuits for one social worker who would, hopefully, solve all of their social problems. Seebohm pointed to growing problems in the way social services were delivered and pointed to poor coordination between social agencies. Now the aim was to bring together all the work of children's departments, the whole of the work of welfare departments and the social work elements in health, education and housing departments (10).

For one former Children's Officer, Tom White, who went on to build Coventry's highly successful and innovative social services department, and to be the first appointed director of social services, Seebohm represented a real change from Poor Law attitudes, on which social services had been based. "There was recognition that tackling entrenched social problems involved 'draining the swamp' – rather than pulling people out . . . Help should be available to ensure communities, particularly in deprived areas, were strengthened and became mutually supportive" (11, p. 177).

Another former Children's Officer, Barbara Kahan, argued that the expansion of Children's Departments, in the 20 years of their existence, into work with families and offenders, meant that its staff were already becoming social workers rather than child care officers. In a statement that has considerable resonance in this book, Kahan argued that a families' difficulties were often associated with housing shortages, policies in allocating housing, social security limits and similar areas of social problems (12). As we shall later explore, however, the location of the new social services departments more centrally in local authorities did not mean that other departments could always mesh more closely than previously, to create a seamless service. At the time of the Seebohm proposals, there was also an articulated fear that these new departments would be run by Medical Officers of Health and subsumed under healthcare services. This represents an interesting perspective given the thinking in recent years that health and social services should now come together.

Recent major changes to health and education

The final shortlist of major landmarks that have affected children's services today is slightly different. So far, we have considered the transformation of education for children, through the 1944 Education Act, the establishment of the NHS, social services (via Children's Departments) and the transformation of welfare benefits, through the 1948 National Assistance Act. Those changes that flowed from both the Boer War and the Second World War were the result of national crises and as such gained a degree of political consensus that worked across the major political parties. Further and major changes considered in the remainder of the chapter have a slightly different provenance. They have largely sprung from one political party, very much in line with a specific ideology and, in the case of education outlined below, modified by subsequent governments. Major policy changes that have swept through the NHS, education, social services, the probation service and the voluntary sector will all be considered in so far as they have fundamentally affected the way we support children and provide a background for later discussion about integrated care.

The 2012 Health and Social Care Act, the so-called "Lansley proposals" after the then Secretary of State for Health, had, to some extent, been trailed by the 1989 White Paper, *Working for Patients* (13). Both were the products of a Conservative government keen to foster competition and open up markets to a wider range of possible providers. The White Paper had at its heart two principles: to give patients better healthcare and greater choice and to generate greater satisfaction and reward for those working in the NHS. Turned into legislation in the 1990 National Health Service and Community Care Act, it allowed hospitals to apply for self-governing status, established the principle that money would follow the patient across administrative boundaries and permitted GP practices to apply for their own budgets to procure services from hospitals. It was also positive about the role the private sector could play in providing services.

The 1989 White Paper introduced what was to become known as the internal market and a new division between those who purchased and those who provided NHS services. How this was to work in practice was that the NHS would decide what care it wanted and then purchase it from self-governing hospitals – known as NHS trusts. To some extent, hospitals were "competing" for patients and it was hoped that this new element of competition would lead to increases in efficiency. GPs were encouraged to become "fund-holders", taking a cash budget for their patients, in order to be able to buy a range of care. Significantly, they could buy from whoever they wished, not just from other NHS providers, but from the private and voluntary sectors. Competition and a more market-driven NHS began to change the health landscape irretrievably.

But the subsequent Health and Social Care Act 2012 was to pursue these earlier changes much further. It abolished what were known as Primary Care Trusts and the Strategic Health Authorities that had responsibility for large geographic areas and the ability to move money from wealthy to cash-strapped trusts.

Now the commissioning of healthcare funds was to be put in the hands of Clinical Commissioning Groups (CCGs), run principally by GPs. They, as primary care providers, were seen by the Secretary of State as being the closest to knowing what local services were required. The Act had three key principles – putting patients at the centre of the NHS, changing the emphasis of measurement to clinical outcomes and empowering health professionals (especially GPs) located within communities. The King's Fund described these proposals as "the biggest re-organisation in the 63 years history of the NHS" (14, p. 10) opening the way for competition, the growth of the private sector in healthcare and what was clumsily described as the "marketization" of the NHS. As one bemused commentator had it, the changes were so big they could be seen from space. And so health trusts were free to go out to contract and compete for work, sometimes in other parts of the country from which they originate and bring in new private providers. As a consequence they have rapidly been compelled to learn about tendering for healthcare.

The merits or drawbacks of this system are not the focus of this book. What remains important to present arguments is that this new and sometimes highly complex commissioning process has seen the NHS move to where other public services, namely education, local government, probation and the voluntary sector, had also been travelling. To some extent these changes occurred later to the NHS than they did to other public services, possibly because of an inherent fear that change could be seen as privatisation and the eventual abandonment of an iconic organisation, loyally and traditionally endorsed by all of the major political parties and certainly by the general public. It is important to understand these changes and the journey towards multiple providers, in terms of later arguments as to how services might be better configured to meet the needs of children and young people. We need to start from an understanding of how the NHS has opened its doors to multiple providers.

If we turn to education, we see a similar journey from largely single providers to a variety of ways in which schools could be organised. The transformation in education and the way that schools are run was, perhaps surprisingly, initiated by a Labour government. It was David Blunkett who, as Secretary of State for Education under Tony Blair, passed the Learning and Skills Act 2000 (15), which established a new learning and skills council and permitted the development of new academies, in order, as Blunkett asserted, to improve pupil performance and to break the cycle of low expectations. The status of becoming an academy was offered to former local authority-maintained schools, with the intention of giving more freedom of autonomy to schools and a greater diversity in the range of provision. They were to remain publicly funded, free from local authority control and with no obligation to follow the National Curriculum (16). Interestingly, the subsequent coalition government passed the Academies Act 2010, which, rather than scrap the legislation of a former administration, widened the scope of academies. It made it possible for all publicly funded schools in England to become academies. They remained publicly funded but with an increased degree of autonomy, such as setting teachers' salaries and moving away from the National Curriculum.

This, and the 2011 Education Act, removed the former requirement for academies to have a specialization in one or more specific subject areas, such as sport or languages. What has happened has been a gradual widening of the range of schools, now including free schools, multi-academy trusts, the self-improving school system, studio schools and university technical colleges Not only is there a greater diversity in schools, but a new freedom for academies to be run by charities, universities, independent schools, community and faith groups, teachers, parents and also businesses. They are funded directly by government and not the local council and often derive funding and sponsorship from a range of sources.

Juvenile justice

Readers will quickly discern a pattern in the way that public services have been evolving. A dropping of restrictions as to who can deliver care for children, whether in health, social care or education, is accompanied by a growth in competition and an opening up of markets to both the private and voluntary sectors. Nowhere is this more in evidence than in the policies of criminal justice reform. Two areas, in particular, stand out. The first of these is usually referred to as offender management services and the second, prison and probation organisation. Following a consultation paper on rehabilitation, the Government introduced a strategy for reform (17) and from 2015 onwards, a large part of the probation service in England and Wales was outsourced to other providers. The existing probation trusts were replaced by a significantly smaller National Probation Service – dealing with high-risk public cases. Supervision of services to offenders assessed as low and medium risk was to be contracted out to a range of providers on a payment by results basis. So, once again, we see markets opened to a diverse range of new – in this case rehabilitation – providers, including existing public but also voluntary and private sector providers. There was also to be a new payment incentives for market providers, in order, as the 2013 reform strategy had it "to focus relentlessly on reforming offenders" (17, n.p.).

Second, the privatisation of some prisons has been no less radical. This was made possible by the 1991 Criminal Justice Act, which led to a combination of newly built private prisons and some, where private companies took over from the prison authorities. In 2017 there were 14 privately run prisons, operated by three companies (about 15% of the countries prisons) and including secure training centres for young people. The principle that prisons might be run by private sector companies can again be compared with the way in which private sector providers now run NHS and other previously state services.

Lastly, in terms of the transformation of services, the chapter needs to acknowledge the sea change in the delivery of voluntary sector services. This has been so fundamental and is now so important in the delivery of services for children, that it will be considered in detail in Chapter 6. In many ways, the voluntary sector also helps to understand the ebb and flow of state and other providers of children's public services.

What this chapter demonstrates is the growing diversity of major providers of services to children and young people. Reforms introduced before the onset of the First World War and even more fundamentally those implemented after the Second, hugely increased the power of the state to care for children's health, education, or social care needs. But, more recently, this monopoly of care, by the State has been replaced by a widening of markets and a greater range of providers. Today, there is considerable diversity as to where care for children might be provided. The efficiency of some of the new models of care is fiercely debated. For all of those who argue that greater competitiveness brings lower costs and greater attempts to measure effectiveness are others who argue that the profit motive is sometimes put before quality and that diversification makes it more difficult for children to receive an holistic service. In other words, a multitude of providers makes it easier to fall between the cracks. The significance of all of this for the book is that any proposals for change, in order to aim at more integrated care for children, must firstly take account of what is now often referred to as the "mixed economy" of care.

Notes

1 *British society 1914–45.* Stevenson, J., 1984, Allen Lane, London.
2 *The fourth revolution.* Micklethwaite, J. and Wooldridge, A., 2014, Penguin Random House, St Ives.
3 Quoted in *Child welfare. England. 1872–1989.* Hendrick, H., 1994, Routledge, London.
4 *The next welfare settlement, Beveridge at 70.* Harrop, A., 2012, The Fabian Society, London.
5 *A prize worth fighting for, Beveridge at 70.* Byrne, I., 2012, The Fabian Society, London.
6 *The road to 1945. British politics and the Second World War.* Addison, P., 1975, Jonathan Cape, London.
7 *Champions for children. The lives of modern child care pioneers.* Holman, B., 2001, The Policy Press, Bristol.
8 *Whose children?* Hurtwood, Lady Allen of, 1945, Hurtwood House, Guildford.
9 I am indebted to Warwick University Library, Modern Records Centre. *Whose children?* Memorandum of evidence submitted to the Care of Children Committee (Curtis Committee) by Lady Allen of Hurtwood, Hurtwood House, Guildford, Surrey, June 1945.
10 *Report of the Committee on Local Authority and Allied Personal Social Services.* 1968, HMSO, Cmnd, 3703, London.
11 *The surprise of my life.* White, T., 2010, Heathcote House, Oxfordshire.
12 *Champions for children.* Holman, B., 2001, The Policy Press, Bristol.
13 *Working for patients.* Department of Health, 1989, HMSO, London.
14 *Never again? The story of the Health and Social Care Act 2012.* Timmins, N., 2012, The King's Fund Institute for Government, London.
15 *Learning and Skills Act.* Department of Education, 2000, HMSO, London.
16 An interesting alternative take on the Labour Party education reforms can be found in Chris Mullin's diary. He quotes a letter from David Blunkett setting out Labour's proposals "Beacon and Specialist schools small Education Action Zones, school-based city learning centres; learning mentors and enriched opportunities for gifted and talented children". Mullin's comment on this is "How about this for a piece of New Labour claptrap". *A view from the foothills*, Mullin, C., 2009, Profile Books, London.
17 *Transforming rehabilitation. A strategy for reform*, Ministry of Justice, 2013, HMSO, London.

3

THE TROUBLED AND TROUBLESOME

Short-term schemes for children

Troubled families

Between 6 and 11 August 2011 riots took place starting in London and then in other major English cities. Demonstrations began in Tottenham, following the shooting and death of Mark Duggan by the police, and resulted in thousands taking part in violence, looting and arson. David Cameron, the then prime minister, decided to launch a programme aimed at families facing multiple challenges. It was based on earlier Cabinet Office analysis of a cohort of families who had numerous needs and often absorbed considerable resources from a range of statutory agencies. Here was an opportunity to move from reactive services to a way of offering early intervention.

The programme to help families facing multiple challenges or "The Troubled Families Programme", as it became known, was to focus on households that had at least three serious problems, such as youth crime or anti-social behaviour, children who regularly truanted or an adult out of work and on benefits. However, Louise Casey, the civil servant who became responsible for developing the scheme, claimed that, on average, targeted families had nine significant problems (1).

Launched with the Department of Communities and Local Government, the fund was given an initial budget of £448 million, with a remit to work with the 120,000 intractable families who were calculated to cost the taxpayer £9 billion a year – of which £8 billion was spent reacting to issues and £1 billion trying to tackle them. It was based on the premise that this relatively small number of families was known to all of the statutory agencies, like the police and social services, and absorbed a disproportionate range of resources.

It was to be a "payment by results" programme. So, the ability of local authorities to turn families round by, for example, finding work for the unemployed or reducing antisocial behaviour would release extra money. So authorities had strong incentives to declare successes. It would not escape the thinking of local authorities that one way of achieving success and accessing the extra funding could lie in aiming to eradicate some of the easier examples of social problems.

In 2013, at the halfway stage of the project, a report from the Department of Communities and Local government (2) claimed that the scheme was on track for success. The report showed that 18 months into the three-year programme over 62,000 families were being worked with and over 22,000 had been turned around. By which was meant that children were back at school, levels of youth crime and anti-social behaviour significantly reduced and over 1,400 adults from some of England's hardest-to-help households were now in continuous work.

However, a report from the National Audit Office, again in 2013, was far less positive (3). Its findings revealed that designing a national programme to support families had potential benefits, but was equally challenging, given a lack of national data. The report argued that not only had the Department of Work and Pensions failed to establish how progress measures would contribute to the programme's outcomes, but that there was only limited understanding of how local authorities would respond to a payment by results scheme. Second, that there was a "potential tension" between definitions of success, shared by the Department of Communities and Local Government. Third, and a criticism levelled at the scheme later, was that the system of payment by results encouraged councils to classify minor complaints, such as excessive noise, as evidence of being a troubled family; so that they were more likely to turn the family round. (The suggestion raised above.) The real fear was that the scheme was not cost effective, was not able to manage the large variations in performance between local authorities and that evidence to evaluate effectiveness needed to be improved. As the 2013 National Audit Office report recorded (p. 10) "early indications also suggest that the incentives may not work in the way that the Departments envisaged".

The Troubled Families Programme is described in some detail because it illustrates some crucial messages about the way central government policies for children and young people evolve. All policy, as we shall explore in greater detail, is driven by a combination of events, expediency and the political philosophy of those in power. As we have already noted, the failure of young men in the Boer War to meet the physical expectations of solders, for example, led to the Liberal reforms of the early twentieth century. With Troubled Families, the 2011 riots had led to a quick response from a government keen to demonstrate it could address social problems with decisive action. What inevitably has altered in the last few years is the speed of change and the necessity of late twentieth and early twenty-first century administrations to match the rapidity at which news and public opinion starts to evolve.

Furthermore, one message from the National Audit Office's analysis of Troubled Families – that the criterion for success was not properly defined or evaluated – is one to which we will return. A second message is that Troubled Families largely saw the responsibility for implementing the scheme lying with local authority social services departments. There was little of the integrated approach to children's problems, which will be explored much more in this book. The very strong financial incentive to succeed was aimed exclusively at stretched local government coffers.

But Troubled Families is just one example of a pattern we will see frequently. This chapter will explore the relationship between policy and political ideology, as it has affected children in the last 20 years, and the way that this is not linked to any rigorous framework of research and evaluation to which, in relation to Troubled Families, the National Audit Office directly alluded. A distinction will be drawn between major initiatives, which have attempted to change the landscape of children's services, and more minor government-inspired changes, which often point to the subtle differences in political ideology. Lastly, reference will also be made to some recent initiatives that have tried to integrate or join up more than one government department or service.

Examples of short-term government initiatives in social care

To begin with, if we turn to short-term initiatives aimed at children and young people some have a symbolic political importance as well as aiming to improve their lives. In 2007, for example, towards the latter years of the Blair/ Brown governments, the Department for Children, Schools and Families was created with a bright rainbow logo and a policy to affect the lives of all young people up to the age of 19. It followed the demerger of the Department of Education and Skills, lasted until 2010 and reflected a more long-standing debate – still very much relevant – as to where children belonged at a central government level. Writing in 2017 in the Parmoor lecture, Sir James Munby captured this when he wrote that there was a division of responsibilities across Whitehall between different departments in matters affecting families and children.

> The Department for Education, the Ministry of Justice, the Department of Health, the Home Office, the Department of Work and Pensions, the Department of Communities and Local Government . . . all have roles to play. It is an intriguing commentary on how Whitehall is organised that there is no Department and no Secretary of State whose title includes either the word "families" or the word "children", though there is a junior Minister, the Minister of State for Children and Families in the Department of Education.
>
> *(4, p. 5)*

Although this book's focus is very much on the lack of integration at a local level, further reference will be made to the way that central government, as Sir Martin Munby illustrates, fails to connect policy. Needless to say, following a general election and change of government in 2010, the rainbow logo disappeared, and the Department of Education was re-instated; re-emphasising the centrality of education rather than social care in the new coalition government's thinking.

What David Cameron, the then prime minister, did announce, however, in 2014, was the "family test", which was to ensure that government policy was to be tested in all departments for its impact on the family. He argued that every government department was to be held to account for the effect of their policies on the family. However, faced with some internal resistance, the scheme was quietly dropped. Writing in *The Sunday Times*, in 2016, Ian Duncan Smith asserted that, two years after its launch the family test had yet to be properly applied (5).

A look at a few of the short-term interventions, which have taken place between 1997 and the present day, helps to illustrate how far services for children have been led by unsustained proposals. This period embraces the Labour governments under Prime Ministers Tony Blair and Gordon Brown (1997–2007) and the Conservative/Liberal Democrat coalition (2010–15), under David Cameron. This list of short-term projects is by no means exhaustive, but encapsulates major developments for children across social care, education and health.

A consistent theme across governments has been the common aim both to intervene early in the lives of families and children, in order to prevent further problems and, through targeted services, offer a combination of education and training. The amount of "education" involved in these projects and the way that this is delivered is very much a reflection of the political hue of the government in power.

One early initiative of the Labour government, in 1997, was the establishment of the Social Exclusion Unit, set up to coordinate central and local government policy-making on specific cross cutting topics, such as school exclusion and truancy, mental health, rough sleeping, teenage pregnancy and young people at risk. One aim was to change the way social exclusion was understood within government; arguing that issues facing teenage parents, rough sleepers and young people are complex and interconnected. It had three aims and reached for solutions based on:

- preventing social exclusion;
- making some mainstream services deliver for everyone;
- reintegrating people who have fallen through the net.

Of course, the work was not exclusively in the area of children and young people, although across the 50 reports published by the Unit, many aimed at addressing social exclusion amongst the younger end of the population.

There was to be a new link between the economics of care and social policy itself. "Joined up solutions to joined up problems" was to be the mantra (6). Followed by the Social Exclusion Task Force, it was abolished by the Coalition government in November 2010 and its functions absorbed into the Office for Civil Society.

This new connection between the economics and social policy aspect of services for children can be found in the Government's Green Paper, *Children First: A New Approach to Child Support*, calling for a radical reform of the child support system and published a year after the establishment of the Social Exclusion Unit (7). It aimed to replace the existing child support system, which was increasingly seen as over complicated and difficult to administer effectively, with a simplified system. All children, it argued, have the right to support from their parents, wherever they may be living. By improving the operation of the child support system, it was also hoped to encourage parental responsibility.

As a further example of a government keen to lose no time in implementing changes to the lives of children and their families, the Home Office published a consultation document in 1998 titled *Supporting Families* (8). It, in turn, took as its starting point the clear principles that the interests of children are paramount, that they need stability and security and the state can better support children rather than trying to substitute for parents. This approach concentrated on five areas

- access to advice and support for parents, including the proposal for a National Family and Parenting Institute;
- financial support including Child Benefit, Working Families Tax Credit and an Education Maintenance allowance;
- helping families balance work and home life with various family-friendly employee arrangement and employee practices;
- strengthening marriage and reducing the risks of family breakdown;
- tackling serious family problems such as truancy and exclusions, youth offending, teenage parenthood and domestic violence.

From this ambitious agenda was born the National Family and Parenting Institute with funding both from government sources and the Joseph Rowntree Foundation. As another example of the vagaries of government policy, the Institute was eventually merged with the Day Care Trust in 2013 and renamed the Family and Childcare Trust.

A landmark initiative, under the Labour government in 2003, was the launch of *Every Child Matters* (9). This, as is acknowledged in the preface to the report, was partly in response to the death of Victoria Climbié in 2000, at the hands of her guardians. Her death, like that of Maria Colwell in 1973, captured the public's attention in a way that separated both tragedies from the sad roll call of other similar child deaths. Not only did the Labour government issue a formal response to Lord Laming's inquiry, set up to investigate Victoria's death (10) but picked up a range of recommendations both in *Every Child Matters* and in the 2004 Children Act that followed.

The aim was to ensure a new emphasis on child protection, making sure all children were to:

- Stay safe
- Be healthy
- Enjoy and achieve
- Make a positive contribution
- Achieve economic well-being.

All children up to the age of 19 were included (24 years old for those with disabilities) with a range of new services incorporated from *Every Child Matters* and the 2004 Children Act. These included a new Director of Children's Services post in each local authority, a lead member for children, in the councils, a new Local Safeguarding Children's Board, again in each locality, a Minister for Children, Young People and Families and the establishment of a Children's Commissioner (see below). Also introduced was a Children's Workforce Development Council and a Sector Skills Council for Children and Young People. In Scotland a similar review *Getting It Right for Every Child* (11) was linked to a review of the Scottish Children's Hearing system, through which children and young people giving cause for concern are referred for help.

Victoria Climbié died in 2000, but the previous year the government had produced *Working Together to Safeguard Children* (12). Basically, it provided statutory guidance, which outlined how practitioners working with children, young people and families should work together. It was subsequently reviewed and re-issued in 2006 and there were three further updates in 2010, 2013 and 2015 – the last focusing on the need for early help. Statutory guidance of this kind does manage to escape the vagaries of new governments, but each iteration tends to reflect the ideology of the administration in power.

Returning to *Every Child Matters*, one of the most significant assertions, which also fits in with a major theme of this book, was that:

> for the first time ever requiring local authorities to bring together in one place under one person services for children.
>
> *(9, p. 9)*

This was also to result in Children's Trusts, discussed later in the chapter. The overall vision in *Every Child Matters* came close to advocating an integrated service bringing together a range of agencies. Nevertheless, the Conservative–Liberal Democrat government of 2010 moved away from this concept and terminology, replacing the five promises, outlined above, with an agreement to "help children achieve more" and a new emphasis on choice for children via tax credits, rather than centrally funded solutions. Again, we see a change of political ideology overturning what was previously seen as innovation.

Both the Children's Workforce Development Council and the Social Care, Children and Young People's Sector Skills Council, established by the then Labour government, aimed to ensure that people working with children had the right skills. The Workforce Council attempted to improve outcomes for children and young people by enhancing the role of the workforce – through training, career development and improved staff mobility. It promoted the training needs for everyone whose work was mainly with children, young people and families. Again, in March 2012, under the relatively new Conservative–Liberal Democrat Coalition, it was closed. Its remit was to work very much in tandem with the Sector Skills Council for Children and Young People, committed to improve productivity and performance statistics, boost skills and improve opportunities for learning. Here, a gradual transformation in the work of the Council resulted in it losing its *Every Child Matters* focus.

Bucking the trend of those short-term initiatives that get quickly replaced with a change of government or minister, has been the establishment of a Children's Commissioner: another recommendation in Lord Laming's Climbié report (10). Wales had established such a post in 2001, Northern Ireland in 2003, Scotland in 2004 and England followed in 2005. Initially established to represent the views and interests of children and young people, the emphasis later changed more to protecting and promoting children's rights. The fact that this initiative has weathered several changes of government is perhaps due to the growth of interest internationally in both children's rights and the flexibility of the role to adapt and mould into differing governments' priorities. The Children's Commissioner role is not so much about the delivery of services, but more about how effective that delivery is, pushing for change and asking the difficult questions.

Enough evidence has been provided to indicate that while the Labour governments between 1997 and 2010 represented a period of intense activity in the field of social care, many of these initiatives were eventually overthrown by a change of political administration. The last example of this was the Centre for Excellence and Outcomes in Children and Young People's service (C4EO), launched in 2008 and originally funded by the Department for Children, Schools and Families. Its aim was partly to assist Children's Trusts in improving outcomes for children – a kind of best practice hub for "what works" in children's services, identifying and coordinating local, regional and national evidence of "what works". As such, it specialised in areas including adoption, children in care, early intervention, safeguarding, special educational needs and disability. Between 2008 and 2011 it operated independently, eventually moving to the National Children's Bureau, working alongside the work of its research centre. This particular initiative takes us closer to one of the book's later explored other themes about the need for research and evaluation in the way services evolve.

A change of government and child care focus

The arrival of the coalition government of Conservatives and Liberal Democrats in 2010 led to a marked shift in initiatives affecting children and young people. One strong strand in the thinking of this new government was the belief in early intervention, coupled with support and encouragement without the need for direct government involvement. The example of the Early Intervention Foundation and the subsequent CANparent scheme, not only highlights this difference of approach from the previous administration but again sadly demonstrates the short-term nature of much centrally driven change.

In 2010 the Prime Minister, David Cameron, had asked MP Graham Allen to chair an independent review into early childhood intervention, which was to report back to the government. From this the Early Intervention Foundation was conceived, born in 2013 with the help of some start-up funding of £3.5 million and cast adrift as an independent charity, later the same year. It was very much based on the belief that addressing a problem's root causes, rather than reacting to its symptoms, would produce better outcomes and would therefore be more cost effective in the long run. Its aim was to evaluate what works and what doesn't work in the areas of early intervention for both programmes and innovative local practice. As a charity, the Foundation linked with other "What works" initiatives, which the government hoped would both influence and change practice.

From this work in the area of early intervention, the CANparent scheme was born in 2012. Launched as an initiative from the Department of Education, CANparent sought to trial an offer of high quality, stigma-free parenting classes to support the enhancement of parenting skills and confidence. The second part of the scheme was to stimulate a commercial market and prevent the need for further, costly intervention. So it aimed at cultivating a quasi-market model, with the classes being offered by a range of private sector providers.

These parenting classes were aimed at parents and carers of children aged 0–5 who qualified for free vouchers, entitling them to attend a course of parenting classed by one of several approved suppliers in their area. The class providers could, in turn, redeem the vouchers at £100 each from the Department of Health. To obtain vouchers, the scheme set up a number of outlets including Boots, GP practices and health centres. The classes themselves were provided in face-to-face groups, 1:1 support, online and self-directed or through a combination of written material plus CD/DVDs. Held in two separate phases, between 2012 and 14 and 2014 and 2015 CANparent was trialled in three English districts (the High Peaks, Derbyshire, Middlesbrough and Camden) with a comparator in Bristol. For the first phase parents were given the £100 voucher for each eligible child. It was hoped to attract 20,000 families, but only reached 2,956. For the second phase, numbers were reduced to 164. Perhaps this was a reflection of the withdrawal of vouchers (13). The final report recognised the value of parenting classes but inevitably raised questions about the continuance of the scheme with no vouchers nor any expectation that either parents themselves or other organisations would help pick up the costs of such a scheme.

To some extent, CANparent was in touch with the zeitgeist. Between 2004 and 2013 there had been a Channel 4 television series, *Shameless*, built around a fictional and feckless family, the Gallaghers, situated in Chatsworth, a housing estate in Manchester. Living very much on the edge, they were presided over by a patriarchal unemployed alcoholic, Frank, who had been left by his wife and abnegated responsibility for bringing up the five siblings to Fiona, their eldest sister. There was a wider public debate about the challenging role of parenting in modern British society, with television programmes looking at the problems on sink estates or the televised intervention of child care experts to quell unruly behaviour and tantrums in young children.

In line with Conservative policies, the Coalition government aimed less at whole-scale intervention and more towards pilot developments focused on specific issues. A good example of this was the Public Health Minister, Anna Soubry, announcing a Department of Health grant of £5.1 million in 2013, in order to get children and families exercising more. Of this, £3 million was awarded to Change4Life Sports Clubs and £1 million for walking initiatives in eight major English cities. The remaining fifth was to be devoted to street play, to revive hopscotch and hide and seek on the streets, helping residents to close roads periodically in order to make the games possible. Here, the impetus was the growing acknowledgement that children were achieving less physical exercise and therefore obesity amongst young people was a growing problem.

But the other side of this is the argument that government initiatives are often not joined up and in some case are little short of becoming contradictory. A Freedom of Information request revealed that since 2010 and 2014 one in three councils had removed some staffed and unstaffed play provision. There had been a 38.9% fall in councils' overall spending on play between 2010 and 2013 and, in terms of adventure playgrounds, one in six facilities had closed since 2010 (14). In order to halt the decline (largely the result of pressure to build new houses), it was calculated that £100 million would be needed to halt the 2014 playgrounds closed between 2014/15 and 2015/16 (15). And, finally, in relation to play space for children, a Labour government's investment of £235 million in developing play facilities through its Play Pathfinders and Play Builders schemes was frozen by Michael Gove when he became education secretary.

Two final initiatives, both implemented by the Coalition government, again demonstrate how a change of government can also lead to a very different direction for services. The first of these was the Life Chances strategy aimed at boosting the life chances of the poorest children in the country, launched in January 2016 and quietly dropped in December of the same year. It was to include measures designed to address child poverty, expand parenting provision and, in a moment of déjà vu, potentially introduce a voucher scheme for parenting classes. Instead, the government promised it would bring forward a social justice green paper, which would incorporate ideas from the original initiative.

A second proposal, which, to some extent represented the Coalition government's move away from Labour's *Every Child Matters* agenda was the proposal to transform children's departments into trusts (a parallel development to the growth of academies in the education sector). This was partly driven by what were seen as failing children's departments and partly a political desire to take some services away from local government control. It found a fuller expression in *Putting Children First*, a policy document launched by the Conservative government in 2016 (16).

Putting Children First outlined a vision for excellent children's social care. The aim was to ensure all vulnerable children, no matter where they lived, would receive the same high quality of care and support. It was built on what were described as the "three pillars" of the social care system, aimed at:

- people and leadership – raising the standards of entry in social work;
- practice and systems – improving data collection and developing a new framework for inquiries into cases of harm to children; and
- governance and acceptability – where the idea of Children's Trusts were more fully explored.

Not only did the document encourage bids for Innovation Programme funding but encouraged new organisational models, including trusts, for the delivery of children's services. It was proposed that this could happen in one of two ways, with children's social care functions delegated to new not-for-profit organisations, separate from local authorities, or by combining authorities across a wider geographical area. The document asserted that by 2020 over a third of current local authorities would either be delivering their children's services through a new model or be actively working towards such a model.

All of this demonstrates that across social care, as for health and education, new service delivery models are evolving and plans for integrated services need to take account of this rapidly shifting landscape.

Before moving on to changes in the way health is delivered, it is worth noting the example of an initiative that has straddled more than one administration. Adoption provides an interesting case study in that both Tony Blair and David Cameron expressed a wish to improve adoption services. Tony Blair revealed a personal connection, as his father, Leo, had been adopted after his travelling entertainer parents left him with a couple they met on tour. In 2000 he launched a White Paper on adoption, *Adoption a New Approach* (17) which, amongst other things promised a 40% increase in adoptions by 2004–5. Inevitably, this led to a temporary surge in the number of adoptions, which was neither sustained nor reached the 40% target.

Similarly, in 2015 David Cameron, then prime minister, said he wanted to speed up the process of adoption. There was he said, no more pressing issue for government than adoption. In 2016 he unveiled an overhaul of the care system, which referenced changes to adoption law, including calls for adoptions to be speeded up and plans for regional adoption agencies. There was a total number of 5,360 adoptions in 2015, (an increase in the total of 3,100 in 2011), which then fell by 12% in 2016 and a further 8% in 2017 to 4,350. At the same time there has been a steady increase in the number of children in care from 60,000 in England in 2009 to 72,670 on 31 March 2017 (18). This increase in children in care is largely attributed to the child protection tragedies and increased vigilance or defensive practice (depending on your viewpoint) from social care agencies.

Adoption is a small but important piece of the child care jigsaw, bringing permanence and stability to children in the care system. However, the messages from this example are salutary. When an area of child care has the prime minister's imprimatur there will be some improvement, albeit time limited. But this short-term initiative that accompanies the surge in numbers is unlikely to prove lasting. None of the initiatives has been sustainable. In the case of adoption and very poor services over a number of years there is now a strong case for arguing that permanent change will only come about through a national adoption agency, with national standards, reports to parliament and a nationwide sharing of data on both adoptees and those children awaiting placements.

Changes in health

So far, ideas for the transformation of services for children and young people have been confined to social care. But during the same period, from the election of the first Blair government to the present day, we have seen the same range of usually short-term innovations in both health and education. Reference has already been made, in Chapter 2, to what became known as the Lansley proposals in health, through the 2012 Health and Social Care Act, introducing Clinical Commissioning Groups and transforming the way healthcare was delivered. Two further initiatives for children and young people deserve consideration: the National Services Framework for Children and Maternity Services and developments around the Child and Adolescent Mental Health Services (CAMHS).

A major health initiative for children in the Labour government of 2001–5 was the launch of the 2004 National Services Framework for Children, Young People and Maternity Services by the Department of Health (19). It was a ten-year plan, again following on from *Every Child Matters*, ambitiously setting standards for the first time for children's health and social care and intending to stimulate long-term and sustained improvement in child health. The Framework aimed to represent a shift with services being designed and delivered around the needs of the child and not just the illness. It began with five key standards:

1. Promoting health and well-being, identifying needs and intervening early;
2. Supporting parenting;
3. Child, young person and family centred services;
4. Growing up into adulthood;
5. Safeguarding and promoting the welfare of children and young people,

and later developed standards for maternity services, children and young people in hospitals, those with complex health needs and mental health issues. A National Service Framework in Wales was also launched a year later in 2005.

These standards required services to give children, young people and their parents increased information and choice of treatment, to introduce a new child health promotion programme, to promote physical health, mental health and emotional well-being by encouraging children and their families to develop healthy lifestyles and to focus on early intervention and tackle health inequalities. Against each of the key standards were markers of good practice, a rationale for their use and guidance on those interventions necessary to meet the standards.

The Framework was seen as a ten-year programme and was important, embracing as it did, not only health and social care, but also the voluntary sector. But, with a change both of government and political philosophy, "must do's" in the Framework turned to aspirations. This repeated pattern of political "short-termism" clearly dominates many of the initiatives outlined in the chapter.

The development of children and adolescent mental health services (CAMHS) demonstrates a similar pattern. The phrase "Cinderella service" remains one of the most frequent clichés in health and social care, but if it does have any currency it is in the area of mental health services for young people. CAMHS were first established in 1995 and by 1998 there were 24 CAMHS innovation projects. They are based on the concept of mental health inter-disciplinary teams, with psychiatrists, psychologists, social workers and therapists offering occupational and family therapy, focused solely on the mental health needs of young people. The services operated at four levels or tiers, similar to Chapter 1's pyramid of need with:

- Tier 1. General advice and treatment for less severe problems by non-mental health specialists;
- Tier 2 CAMHS specialists working in community and primary care, e.g. mental health workers;
- Tier 3 Multidisciplinary teams or services working in a community mental health clinic;
- Tier 4 Highly specialist services, offering, for example, in-patient treatment.

Since the early 1990s there had been a succession of reviews and policy documents focused on commissioned research, advisory groups to governments, independent reviews (20) and the expertise of those working with the National CAMHS support services and subsequently the National Advisory Council for Children's Mental Health and Psychological Wellbeing (both now disbanded organisations).

Back in 1994 a National Review of Services for the Mental Health of Children and Young People highlighted the huge variations in mental illness service development across the UK (21). This was followed by further reviews from the Health Select Committee, the Audit Commission and other public bodies. This led to a process of policy development, policy research and investment in services, which resulted in the formation of CAMHS. Later, the 2012 Health and Social Care Act created new legal responsibilities within the NHS to build what was described as a "parity of esteem" between physical and mental health. The reality is that children's mental health has remained a low priority compared with adult mental health. A number of specific initiatives have also struggled to retain a commissioning expertise, through all of the many organisational and structural changes that have been affected by both the NHS and local authorities (22). As always, service improvements were dependent upon a combination of the level of priority given to children's mental health within wider government policy, targeted investment by both the NHS and local authorities, help from the national CAMHS support service and the findings of research. That this has not happened consistently illustrates a familiar theme in the chapter. Once again, a change of government has usually meant a discarding or watering down of previous policy and new initiatives. (For further examples of short term health initiatives see Note 23).

Changes in education

If we turn to education, the pattern of well-intentioned but short-lived interventions is no less in evidence. Chapter 2 considered the changes introduced by the Labour government of 1997–2001, which permitted the development of new academies and transformed the landscape of R.A. Butler's 1944 Education Act. Subsequent interactions by the Coalition government of 2010–15 reduced the link between local authorities and schools, introduced free schools, run by parents, and, in line with Conservative thinking, developed much further the idea of choice and freedom from local government control.

The Labour governments, from 1997 onwards, were keen to intervene and influence directly what went on in the classroom. In 1998 they introduced Education Action Zones and the National Literacy and Numeracy Strategies. Education Action Zones were based on the Education Priority Areas, drawn up by a previous Labour government in the late 1960s, aiming to provide teachers working in difficult schools with a special allowance in order to address the divergence in standards between average performance and that of pupils in areas of social disadvantage. Their introduction was one of the first actions of the new government, aiming to raise standards in disadvantaged and rural areas so they could become high achievers. They mirrored the Health Action Zones (24), also introduced by New Labour in 1998 in 15 areas – another intervention aimed at reducing inequality. There were two forms, developed by the Department of Education and Skills, in which the zones were developed – Excellence in Cities Action Zones (EiC) (to address problems in the major conurbations) and Education Action Zones (EAZ) (to bring the same advantage to small pockets of deprivation). By mid-2005 there were 134 Excellence in Cities Action Zones and 80 Education Action Zones. Usually, they linked around 20 schools, consisting of two or three secondary schools and the rest primary schools and nurseries. Subsequent Ofsted reports on their effectiveness were mixed and they were subsumed by fresh initiatives.

If Education Action Zones strove to affect the infrastructure through which education to children was delivered, the National Literacy and Numeracy strategy went straight to the heart of the classroom. This project was the result of a literacy task force set up by David Blunkett in May 1996, while Shadow Education Secretary and under the chairmanship of Professor Michael Barber. What was unusual about this initiative was that it was planning for government well before ministerial office had been won. The aim was to raise children's levels of achievement drastically. In literacy, for example, the aim was that by 2002 80% of 11-year-olds would reach the standard of their age in English (i.e. level 4) in the Key Stage 2 National Curriculum tests. It established a literacy hour where whole class learning on a shared text was to last 15 minutes, whole class focused work on spelling and grammar (15 minutes), independent and guided group work (20 minutes) and whole class reflection on what has been learnt (10 minutes) There was never a numeracy hour in quite the same way, but, again, targets were set for 75% of 11-year-olds reaching the standard of mathematics expected for their age by 2002. Scotland,

Wales and Northern Ireland had their own curricula and education departments were not formally affected by the National Literacy Strategy. There was some initial success and improvements in performance, but sceptics criticised it as not being part of a coherent education strategy and of setting unrealistic national targets.

In relation to both of the above initiatives, a 2014 report, under the aegis of the Institute for Education at the University of London, provided an overall analysis of Labour's educational achievements (25). They concluded that Labour politics led to a small but important reduction in the attainment gap between children from deprived backgrounds and their wealthier peers, although it cannot be said to have matched the government's own aspirations. Policies with credible indicators of a positive impact included the National Literacy and Numeracy Strategies and Extended Schools (see below). Some other policies that practically benefitted disadvantaged children included the one-to-one Reading Recovery intervention and Teach First (26). Interestingly, the report notes that the quality of initiatives launched by Labour – and the tendency to adjust them without robust evaluation – made it difficult to tell which were effective. Evidence on policies such as reduced class sizes, increased use of teaching assistants, Education Action Zones and Excellence in Cities (27) is equivocal at best. The lack of any proper evaluation is serious and one to which we will return at the end of the chapter.

Four further education and training initiatives, which aimed at older children and young people, deserve brief consideration. The Learning and Skills Council, established in 2001, under the Learning and Skills Act 2000 (which looked at post 16 education and training) replaced the 72 Training and Enterprise Councils and the Further Education Funding Council for England. It was a non-departmental public body, jointly sponsored by the Department for Business, Innovation and Skills and the Department for Children, Schools and Families. It was responsible for planning and funding further education (post-16 education) and was at one stage described as Britain's largest quango. It was established so that young people in England would have the knowledge and production skills, leading unashamedly to a world class standard workforce. It lasted until 2010 when the responsibilities were transferred to a new Skills Funding Agency and Young People's Learning Agency.

In a similar vein, New Labour increasingly focused on the delivery of targeted services to those who were often described as most in need of help. They replaced the Careers Service with Connexions, offering support and advice for 13–19-year-olds (and up to 25 for those with learning difficulties and/or disabilities) on education, housing, health, relationships, drugs and finance. The aim was to ensure a smooth transition from compulsory schooling to post-16 learning). As part of the Department of Education and Skills, a network of 47 Connexions partnerships were initially set up, to reduce the number of young people not in education, employment or training, through the recruitment of personal advisers to assist them. Again, the validity of Connexions was eventually called into question; it ceased to be a national service and was dropped by the Conservative/Liberal Democrat coalition government.

As further evidence of this constant churn, the Conservative government established the Careers and Enterprise Company (CEC) in 2015, as a social enterprise, to be the strategic coordinating function for employers, school, colleges and providers – in order to provide careers and enterprise support for young people. It developed a network connecting schools and colleges with employers and careers programme providers, supporting them to work together with the aim of offering effective work experiences for young people. It, in turn, followed on from the National Careers Service, established in 2012 and which originated in a strategy document produced by the Department of Business, Innovation and Skills for everyone over the age of 13. Finally, in what appears to be a tangled landscape of employment activities for young people and adults was Jobcentre Plus, established by the Department for Work and Pensions in 2002 and eventually dissolved in 2011. Formed from the amalgamation of two agencies: the employment service (which operated Jobcentres) and the Benefits Agency, which ran social security offices, its primary task was to help those who were looking for employment and often required financial help because of their lack of employment. As so often is the case with other policies we have seen, differing political ideologies led to differing strategies as to how employment and income support should be organised.

Lastly, and the exception that proves the rule, was the Youth Justice Board established in 1998 but which survived subsequent changes of government. Significantly, in the 1997 Labour Party manifesto was a recognition that the juvenile justice system needed an overhaul and in the following year the Crime and Disorder Act 1998 led to the Youth Justice Board being set up, to establish standards, reduce offending amongst under 18s and manage the youth offending teams. The teams, in their turn, aimed towards integrated services involving social service departments, the police, health, housing, probation, education and drug and alcohol workers. Basically, the Youth Justice Board had three functions, achieved through working through its partners:

- the Youth Offending Teams (YOTs) mentioned above;
- the community youth justice services and their partners;
- the youth secure estate – consisting of youth offending institutions, secure training centres and secure children's homes.

The aim was for the establishment of a Youth Offending Team in each local authority. It was also set up to cover Wales.

That it has survived – albeit as the subject of a number of government cuts – is probably because it provides governments with an overview of youth justice issues across all local authorities. Given, as we saw in relation to Troubled Families and the riots that proceeded this initiative, that youth violence and unrest is a potentially vulnerable issue for all governments, the Youth Justice Board provides a way of monitoring progress and can give an early alert of potential problems.

Proposed change aimed at the integration of services

Enough evidence has been provided to demonstrate that governments enter power with a strong determination to make a difference through policy change. Because of the parliamentary cycle they usually aim for quick fixes. For those administrations fortunate enough to secure a second term this provides an opportunity to strengthen or redefine favourite priorities, usually to be overturned by a new government with a fresh and different set of political ideologies or even a new minister in the same administration. In the last section of this chapter the emphasis will be on those government initiatives that have been driven by a desire to recognise that the future lies in the integration of key services. So change was to be achieved by developing large, overarching strategies that sometimes spanned more than one government department. Here, several major examples will be briefly discussed: Total Place, Extended Schools and the raft of initiatives that resulted in the Children's Fund, Children's Centres and Sure Start initiatives.

Total Place fits firmly in the list of government initiatives aimed at the greater integration of local services. Launched in the Labour government's budget of 2009 it was predicated both on getting local public services to work together and to save money through what was described as "whole system intervention". When initially launched it was hoped to save up to £20 billion in ten years through a combination of pooled budgets and cuts to the duplication of services.

Total Place was wider than the integration of children's services and was formulated as recasting the relationship between local public service organisations – for adults and children – and the centre (28). But, as part of Total Place, local authorities and their Children's Trust partners (see below) could trial a new multi-agency children and young people's grant, to start in April 2011. This grant was to include money for youth activities, school improvement, support for families and disabled children and Sure Start schemes (see below) and would be ring fenced.

Total Place was developed in 13 local authorities, as diverse as Birmingham and Bournemouth and was presented both as a new freedom from central government controls and ability to take a fresh look at what money was coming into a specific area. This was to determine whether it could be more effectively distributed. By its very nature Total Place set up a complicated relationship between central and local government, in order to gauge what savings might be made from taking a "whole area" approach to specific problems or services. It was, however, subsequently dropped by the following administration and partly replaced in 2010 by the Prime Minister, David Cameron's "Big Society" initiative. This, in turn, was launched as giving more power to communities through a combination of devolved powers and localism, the encouragement of people to take an active role in their communities by volunteering, support for co-ops, mutual and social enterprises and the transfer of responsibility from central to local government. This represented a very different approach to that of Total Place, which, at its heart, had a real recognition that what is often described as "silo" working does not succeed and only when services come together can the holistic needs of local communities be best served.

While Total Place, like so many initiatives, was overtaken by a new (in this case coalition) government, the idea of bringing services together emerged in Chancellor George Osborne's announcement in 2014 of a "Northern Powerhouse", which would boost the northern economy by bringing together skills, innovation, transport and culture and by devolving significant powers and budgets to directly elected Mayors. It was specifically targeted at the core northern cities of Manchester, Liverpool, Leeds, Sheffield, Hull and Newcastle, intent on improving transport links and investing in, for example, science and innovation. The similarity with Total Place, although the scale is different, lies in the recognition that bringing services together and building a network of parties who strongly believe in the economic potential of the north would provide a more coherent approach to infrastructure challenges.

More limited than Total Place, but still aiming at the integration of some services for children can be found in the Labour government's Extended Schools initiative. Aimed at building twenty-first-century schools, it arose from Every Child Matters and the Five Years Strategy for Children and Learners. The explicit intention was to improve levels of educational achievement for disadvantaged children and young people, by providing them with additional support. Extended Schools were to offer a range of activities outside of the normal school day. Activities to support learning were to include breakfast or homework clubs, sport, art, drama, ICT programmes for parents and families and the community use of school premises (29).

It began in 61 local authorities in 2003/4 with the aim of reaching all local authorities in 2005/6 – all of them in Behaviour Improvement Programme areas (30).

What is particularly important, in the context of this book is the idea that schools could become hubs of activities into which other organisations would flow. And, of course, schools have the advantage of being a neutral, universal and non-stigmatising resource.

In a pattern that will now be all too familiar to readers, the 2010 Coalition government promised an end to the state monopoly of schools, the growth of academies and extra money for the education of the poorest pupils. As a result, the 2010 Comprehensive Spending Review announced that the amount of Extended Schools funding would be part of the overall schools revenue funding from April 2011. There would be no more earmarked money, as such, for Extended Schools.

Every Child Matters and Children's Trusts

The final section focuses on a series of Labour initiatives originating from the death of Victoria Climbié in 2000. It led, in turn, to Every Child Matters 2003, the 2004 Children Act and Children's Trusts. But another strand that fed into Labour's efforts to address inequality was the publication of the UNICEF report on child poverty 2000 (31). In a survey of 23 rich nations, the UK emerged as 20th out of 23, in terms of children living in relative poverty; just above Italy, the USA and Mexico.

Here, relative poverty is defined as households with an income below 50% of the national median. It led to a broad social programme, starting with Children's Trusts and progressing to the ambitious Sure Start programme.

The Children's Fund was launched in November 2000, as part of the commitment to tackle disadvantage amongst children aged 5–13 years, their families and communities and to make a significant contribution to *Every Child Matters*. It was introduced in three waves from November 2000 to April 2003 and was to operate in each of the 149 local authorities in England, through Children's Fund partnerships and programmes, delivered in schools and community venues. The underlying principles were those of prevention, partnerships and participation. Through an early intervention and multi-agency approach, the programme aimed to identify children at risk of social exclusions and provide necessary support. Two principles – that of early intervention and tackling problems through a range of agencies working together – were core to the scheme and important to this book. Eventually, Children's Fund initiatives were absorbed into Children's Trust arrangements, outlined below. The schemes were to be in partnership with the statutory and voluntary sectors, each working within a local authority area in England.

A cornerstone of Every Child Matters, which initiated some of these Labour initiatives, was the checklist of five key indicators, listed earlier, to drive services – "be healthy, stay safe, enjoy and achieve, make a positive contribution and achieve economic wellbeing" (9, pp. 6–7). Driven by the message that had been repeated in so many child protection tragedies, the Labour government sought to bring departments together. This was to happen through Children's Trusts, which would aim at the integration of organisations responsible for services for children, young people and families in a shared commitment to improving children's lives. Local authorities would be involved, via the children's departments, health, through strategic health authorities and primary care trusts. The police would take part and there would be encouragement from schools and third sector organisations to become involved. The term Children's Trust was applied to the whole system of children's services. There was to be a formal board and the development of local strategies for improving children's lives by delivering better services. The trusts were to aim at specific issues, such as:

- reducing under achievement in early years;
- improving services for disabled children;
- identifying children and young people at risk of failure;
- narrowing the gap – especially in educational attainment between vulnerable children and young people (for example, those in care);
- reduce child poverty.

These were bold aims and the roll out of 35 Pathfinder Children's Trusts had high expectations riding on their coat tails. While trusts were aimed at a co-ordinated local approach to planning for children, there was nothing to prevent services being combined. The expectation was that most areas would have Children's Trusts by 2006 and all by 2008. However, by 2010, following the election of the Conservative and Liberal Democrat Coalition, the requirement on local authorities to set up a Children's Trust board and to prepare a joint children and young people's plan was dropped. Such an approach was assisted by an Audit Commission report, two years earlier, *Are We There Yet* (32), which reported:

> There is little evidence that Children's Trusts, as required by the government have improved outcomes for children and young people or delivered better value for money over and above locally agreed cooperation.
>
> *(p. 65)*

Several themes have a resonance here that also reverberate across a raft of government initiatives. First, as so often seen, a change of policy results in a new direction and a ditching of previous government schemes. Second, as is again often the case, an experiment is abandoned before it has been properly evaluated. (More will be said about the difference, say, between social care and medicine and the way new forms of intervention receive proper evaluation). Third, we see an immediate response from a government wanting to react to public pressure by imposing new structures rather than properly evaluating those that already exist. Children's Trusts represent the closest to an integrated children's service that we have seen in the UK.

The final New Labour initiative, which aimed at integrated services, by basing a range of support in the same location, can be found in the Children's Centre schemes. This eventually became the Sure Start initiative.

Focused on improving outcomes for young children and their families, with a particular emphasis on the most disadvantaged, Children's Centres aimed at reducing inequalities in three ways. As defined by the Department of Education these were:

- child development and school readiness, supported by improved:
- parenting aspirations, self-esteem and parenting skills;
- child and family health and life chances.

(33)

The centres were mostly located in the most deprived areas, with a mix of structured and neighbourhood problems, such as high unemployment or poor housing and individual difficulties including poor health or low self-esteem. The aim was to establish such centres in every deprived community.

The model of delivering centre-based integrated multi-agency services with parental outreach, family support, health services and links to local neighbourhood nurseries and childminders was seen as so successful that the then Labour government decided to develop a network of what became known as Sure Start Children's Centres. These would be universally accessible, not post coded as the Children's Centres had been, but at the heart of every community across the country. In addition, control of children's centres, including funding and commissioning would be passed to local communities. According to the Department of Education (34) Sure Start Centres (building upon what had been learnt from Children's Centres), should be "a place or a group of places", which are managed by or on behalf of or under arrangements with the local authority with a view to securing that early childhood services in the local authority are made available in an integrated way. They should be places:

- through which early childhood services are made available (either by providing the service on site, or by providing advice or assistance on gaining access to services elsewhere); and at which activities for young children are provided;
- like Children's Centres, the core purpose was to improve outcomes for young children and their families and reduce inequalities between families in the greatest need and their peers.

By the time of the report from the All Parliamentary Sure Start Group in July 2013 (35) there were 3,116 centres in England, which ranged from fully integrated "new build" centres, often located on school sites, to small signposting services based in libraries or GP surgeries and reaching 2.7 million children.

As part of the 2010 Comprehensive Spending Review, funding for Sure Start Children's Centres was no longer ring-fenced and became part of the wider Early Intervention Grant. So, by 2014/15, the funding available was calculated to reduce by £0.9 billion. Between 2010 and 2013 about 500 centres shut with 3,631 still open in April 2010 and 3,055 by 2013. Once again, with a change of government and the Coalition Conservative/Liberal Democrat alliance, Sure Start projects were not been given the same priority and the numbers subsequently reduced further. What also stopped was the exploration of a scheme to pool the budgets spent on early years' education (36). Those looking for reasons to close or reduce the Sure Start initiative pointed to some research that indicated that the families and children who were adept at accessing Children's Centre facilities were not necessarily those in greatest need and for whom the centres had been established.

Constant change and a lack of evaluation

To Daniel Defoe's adage that nothing is more certain than death and taxes might be added the short-term initiatives of all political parties. Chapter 2 examined the way in which the Boer War and the Second World War led to social changes that, very unusually, outlasted the normal five-year parliamentary cycle. What characterises so many of the examples examined here, and the list is by no means exhaustive, is the short time that, like firework rockets, they rise, shine and fall. All governments are driven by a desire to make a difference, which inevitably means that they will both discard the policies of the previous administration and reflect the overall tenor of their beliefs in individual "pet" initiatives. This is easily demonstrated by the example of academy schools or the evolution of NHS services, where the ebb and flow of engagement with the private sector is either encouraged or shunned by Labour and Conservative administrations.

So, initiatives are short term, rarely planned in much detail before a new government takes power (although David Blunkett's Numeracy and Literacy Strategy contradicts this general rule) and even more rarely evaluated. For, on top of the imperative of a new government, keen to make its mark on the electorate is the pressure of new and often rapidly replaced government ministers, also wishing to put their stamp on policy. They might crudely be characterised as "hokey cokey" initiatives, just as quickly pulled out, as they are put in.

But, inevitably, whatever blueprints an incoming government may wish to roll out, they are often overtaken by the unforeseen. Harold Macmillan when famously asked what he most feared as prime minister replied, "Events, dear boy events". We have seen how "events", such as the tragic death of Victoria Climbié, the investigation into failed paediatric services in Bristol or the Tottenham riots all led to changes of direction. Governments are always anxious to demonstrate that they are responding both to new pressures and to the wider electorate.

Other writers have pointed to this endless succession of government initiatives. Reference has already been made to the Institute of Education report on New Labour education initiatives to narrow the achievement and participation gaps. Their conclusion that the combination of a large number of initiatives and a tendency to adjust or change them before fully evaluating, is true of all parties (37). A cynical view might lead to the conclusion that policy is driven more by political expediency and the carousel of changing ministerial office, rather than by any thought through evaluation of effectiveness. Writing in his 2010 evaluation of children's health services, Sir Ian Kennedy expressed "a fervent hope" that a:

> new Government could curb the temptation to continue this never ending treadmill of policies. Time and effort would be better spent over the next five years in establishing a clear direction of change . . . and then ensuring that it is actually implemented i.e. that rhetoric becomes reality.
>
> *(38)*

Yet of equal concern is the lack of any rigorous research and evaluation that combines two essential functions. First, to look at the effectiveness of what has been achieved and second to fine-tune this achievement, in order to improve the next iteration of a scheme. It is tempting to ask if the constant wave of initiatives within children's services are replicated in other areas of government. While medicine has a tradition of moving forward based on evidence, this is less the case in areas like youth policy, education or social care. There is, for example, little experience in children's social care of randomised controlled trials, to calculate the effectiveness of an intervention and to estimate the extent to which it achieves more good than harm. Compare this, for example, with the testing of new drugs and medical treatments, where randomised controlled trials are required to prove efficacy or cost effectiveness before they are prescribed by the NHS.

It could be argued that this is a naïve approach and social policy is by its nature driven by that combination of events and political ideology we have outlined above. There are, after all, far more variables in the area of human behaviour which makes proceeding on the basis of hard evidence and the fine tuning of systems difficult. But the consequence of this is that we are often blown by the winds of expediency and political preference. Rather than hold on to those areas of an initiative which seem to work, we are more likely to proceed by simply trumping one scheme with a new one.

As a final example of this latter point, the Parenting Early Intervention Programme (PEIP) provides a salutary lesson. It was set up under a Labour government and between 2008 and 2011 provided government funding to all 150 local authorities, to deliver selected parenting programmes that already had evidence of their efficacy in improving parental outcomes and associated reductions in children's behavioural difficulties. The four main schemes evaluated were Triple P, The Incredible Years, the Strengthening Families Programme 10–14 and Strengthening Families, Strengthening Communities. On completion of the scheme the then Labour government, under the auspices of the Department of Children, Schools and Families commissioned some research on the effectiveness of the programme, which, by the time it delivered its findings, did so to the Department for Education and a new government (39). The results demonstrated that all four of the parenting programmes were effective in improving outcomes for parents and children and these outcomes could still be evidenced one year on from the end of the programme. But, of course, a new government meant a new approach, rather than building on what had gone before.

All of this adds up to a particular challenge for anyone advocating a fundamental change that is both properly evaluated and will probably take 20 years before it can be fully implanted.

Notes

1 *A magnet for trouble: UK's family secret.* Shellen, N., 2014, *The Sunday Times.* 17 August.

2 *Troubled families programme on track at halfway stage.* Department of Communities and Local Government, 2013, HMSO, London.

3 *Programme to help families facing multiple challenges.* National Audit Office, 2013, HMSO, London.

4 *Children across the juvenile justice system.*The 2017 Parmoor lecture to the Howard League for Penal Reform. Sir James Munby.

5 Families are falling apart and the left just wants to stand and watch. Smith, Ian Duncan, Feb. 26, 2017, *The Sunday Times.*

6 *The Social Exclusion Unit.* Office of the Deputy Prime Ministers, 1997, HMSO, London.

7 *Children first: a new approach to child support.* Department of Social Security, Green Paper, 1998, CM 3992, London.

8 *Supporting families: a consultation document.* Home Office, 1998, HMSO, London.

9 *Every child matters.* HM Treasury 2003, Cm, 5860, London.

10 *The Victoria Climbié inquiry.* Report of an Inquiry by Lord Laming, 2003, Cm 5730.

11 *Getting it right for every child. A report on the responses to the consultation on the review of the children's hearing system,* Scottish Government, 2004, Scottish Executive, n.p.

12 *Working together to safeguard children: a guide to inter-agency working to safeguard and promote the welfare of children*. Department of Health, Home Office, Department for Education and Employment, 1999, HMSO, London.
13 *CANparent trial evaluation: phase 2: final report*. Lindsay, G., Cullen, Mm, Cullen, S., Totsika, V., Bakopoulou, I., Brind, R., Chezelayagh, S., Conlon, G., 2016, University of Warwick.
14 Outdoor play under threat from local facilities and funding cull. Jozwiak, G., 2014, *Children and Young People Now*, 7–20 January.
15 Press release. Report of the Association of Play Industries. 13 April 2017, Nowhere to Play campaign.
16 *Putting children first: delivering our vision for excellent children's social care*. Department for Education, July 2016.
17 *Adoption: a new approach*. Department of Health and Social Care, December 2000.
18 *Children looked after in England including adoption: 2016–17*. Department for Education, September, 2017, London.
19 *National Services Framework for Children, Young People and Maternity Services. Core Standards*. Department of Health, 2004, London.
20 I am grateful to Dr Bob Jezzard, formerly professional adviser 1994–2006 for child mental health policy at the Department of Health.
21 *Services for the mental health of children and young people in England: a national review*. Kurtz Z., Thornes, R. and Wolkind, S., 1994, London Maudsley Hospital and South Thames (West) Regional Health Authority, London.
22 See, for example, *Children and young people. Promoting emotional health and well being*. Department of Health, NHS South Central, NHS South East Coast and Care Services Improvement Partnership South East Development Centre, 2008, Department of Health, London.
23 For example, the Labour government launched two further initiatives. In 2008 the *Healthy Child* programme, a public health initiative for children, young people and families which focused on early intervention and prevention and, in the following year *Healthy lives, brighter futures: the strategy for children and young people's health*, Department for Children, Schools and Families, Department of Health, 2009, Department of Health and Department for, Schools and Families, London.
24 Health Action Zones were launched in 1998 in 15 areas followed by a second wave of 11 in 1999. Their focus was on community based activities, to tackle health inequalities
25 *How did New Labour narrow the achievement and participation gap?* Whitty, G. and Anders, J., 2014. Centre for Learning and Life Chances in Knowledge Economics and Societies. Institute of Education, University of London.
26 The Reading Recovery programme is a school based short-term intervention designed for children aged 5 or 6 who are the lowest achieving in learning literacy, after their first year in school. Teach First or Teach First Cymru was founded in 2002 as a social enterprise and registered as a charity, which aimed to address educational disadvantage in England and Wales, by coordinating an employment based teacher training programme. This was achieved by encouraging young graduates to enter teaching, while paying them as soon as they began to practice.
27 Excellence in Cities was launched by the Labour government in 1999 by the Labour government to raise standards and promote inclusion in inner cities and other urban areas. To begin with it targeted secondary schools but was later expanded to include primary schools.
28 *Total place. A practitioner's guide to doing things differently*. Leadership Centre for Local Government, 2010, March, London.
29 *Evaluation of the full service extended schools project: final report*, Cummings, C., Dyson, A., Muijs, D., Papps, I., Pearson, D., Raffo, C., Tiplady, L., Todd, L. and Crowther, D., 2005, University of Manchester and Department for Education and Skills Research Report No 852, London.

30 Behaviour Improvement Programmes were set up in 2002 as part of the Government's Street Crime initiative. In total, 34 authorities were initially chosen to improve poor behaviour and attendance in schools, based on street crime and truancy indicators.
31 *Child poverty in rich nations*. UNICEF, Innocenti Report card, issue no 1, June 2000.
32 *Are we there yet? Improving governance and resource management in Children's Trusts*. Audit Commission, Local Government National Report 2008, London.
33 *Evaluation of children's centres in England. Research looking at the effectiveness of children's centres in England at providing services for eligible families*. Department for Education, June 2014, London.
34 *Sure Start children's centres statutory guidance. For local authorities, commissioners of local health services and JobCentre Plus*. Department for Education, April 2013, London.
35 *Best practice for a Sure Start: the way forward for Children's Centres*, Report for the All Parliamentary Sure Start Group, July 2013, 4Children, London.
36 The idea for pooled budgets for early year's services was explored by the All Party Sure Start group. They argued that separate funding streams created a solo mentality and poor coordination and support. Local authorities' Health and Well Being Boards and their local partners could, it was argued, use pooled budgets to allow for more innovative commissioning of perinatal and children's centre services, permitting what the group described as a more "holistic and preventive" approach to working with families.
37 See also criticism of the *Troubled Families* initiative by the National Audit Office (3) for the scheme's lack of clear evaluation
38 *Getting it right for children and young people. Overcoming cultural barriers in the NHS so as to meet their needs*. Kennedy, Sir Ian, 2010, Department of Health and Social Care, London.
39 *Parenting early intervention programme evaluation*. Lindsay, G., Strand, S., Cullen, M., Cullen, S., Band, S., Davis, H., Conlon, G., Barlow, J. and Evans, R., 2011, Research Report, Department for Education, London.

4

INDICES OF CHILDHOOD

Comparable European data

Born to fail

"We are making progress, but slower than other countries" (1, p. 6). This was one of the conclusions from a 2017 report into the state of child health in the UK from the Royal College of Paediatrics and Child Health (RCPCH). Just like an end-of-term report from the school headmaster, indicating that there had been some improvement, but "could do better" and more was necessary. So far, material presented in earlier chapters has been largely qualitative. We have examined the fractured nature of current children's services, pointed to some gaps and duplications and made reference to the services that have failed children. Reference has also been made to the short-term, politically expedient initiatives of many governments; often knee-jerk reactions to public events, such as the Tottenham riots, the death of Victoria Climbié or the results of a specific political ideology (e.g. the roll-out of academy schools). We have also considered the two or three significant periods in UK history, such as the Boer and Second World War, when changes have been so profound that they have been capable of resisting the vagaries of a new political administration and have rarely outlasted a change of government.

If we have a convincing case that, first, we are failing children in significant ways, second, that some aspects of the lives of children are getting no better or even deteriorating and that, third, in comparison with other similar countries and in accordance with shared measures we are failing, then firmer statistical evidence is needed to support the arguments. This chapter examines a range of measures to provide quantitative evidence on *how* we fail children. It will examine indicators on children's health, statistics on child poverty, education, the protection of children from harm and abuse and, lastly, how children in the care system compare with their peers.

However, several notes of caution are necessary. First, some data have not been collected over a sufficiently long period of time to allow meaningful interrogation. An example of this is the use of the Internet, as a tool to abuse children. Given the comparatively short time in which the Internet has been available, it is difficult to be definitive as to whether this is a growing challenge or static problem. What we do know is that it wasn't a problem 30 years ago, but the overall data are comparatively new to make trends difficult to gauge. Second, where international comparisons might be made, countries sometimes collect data in different ways and this, again, makes any evaluation difficult. Third, no data of this kind is entirely neutral and may be coated by a particular view or argument. Even quantitative data is not value free and care is needed in its interpretation. Vigilance is necessary in the way we handle this material and the conclusions we subsequently draw about the lives of affected children.

In 1973, ten years after the foundation of the NCB, *Born to Fail?* (2) was published, examining the experiences of children. It was based on a large longitudinal study of 16,000 children, all born in the week of 3-9 March 1958 and was multidisciplinary in its scope. A follow up study, *Greater Expectations, Raising Aspirations for our Children* (3), published in 2013 and which was more quantitative in its analysis, took 12 indicators against which children's lives could be evaluated:

- number of children living in poverty;
- proportion of children living in poverty by family circumstances;
- number of children in early education;
- proportion of four-year-olds that achieved a good level of development in the Early Years Foundation stage;
- proportion of 11-year-old pupils achieving the expected level in English and Maths;
- proportion of 16-year-olds achieving five or more A*–C GCSEs;
- absence rates from school – due to illness;
- proportion of children aged 2–15 who are obese;
- proportion of babies born with a low birth weight;
- children living in overcrowded housing or temporary accommodation;
- proportion of UK children aged nine months to three years unintentionally injured at home;
- proportion of children reporting two or more unfavourable environmental conditions.

As is evidenced, from these indicators, they ranged across health, housing and education. Referring back to *Born to Fail?*, *Greater Expectations* records that, in 1973,

> One in seven of those children were growing up in poverty and one in six in poor and overcrowded housing. It also uncovered a clear relationship between growing up in disadvantaged circumstances and the children's outcomes – the inequality in childhood.
>
> *(3, p. 3)*

Furthermore, children living in the most disadvantaged circumstances were, not surprisingly, less healthy and more likely to struggle at school than their more advantaged peers. They were more likely to be born underweight, miss schooling as a result of ill health and to have a high incidence of injuries in the home. They were also less likely than their peers to do well in reading or maths. *Born to Fail?* demonstrated the massive accumulation of additional hardships that confront the most disadvantaged children, in almost every aspect of their daily lives.

Greater Expectations firstly recognized that it is difficult to make comparisons with data from almost half a century ago, due to changing definitions and the existence of differing data sources. Nevertheless, using official sources, the NCB were able to return to the same 12 indices. The report concluded that the number of children in poverty had increased by 1.5 million, since *Born to Fail?* was published and that a child from a disadvantaged background was still far less likely to do well in GCSEs at 16. Furthermore, obesity is more likely in deprived areas and children are more prone to suffer accidental injury at home. Children were also much less likely to have access to green spaces and places to play, if living in deprived areas (3). As the report concluded:

> The fact that the poverty and inequality experienced by our children remains just as prevalent today as it did nearly 50 years ago must not be ignored. Unless a new course of action is taken there is a real risk of sleepwalking into a world where inequality and disadvantage are so deeply entrenched that our children grow up in a state of social apartheid.
>
> *(p. 1)*

This was a strong indictment of inequality in the UK, which deserves exploring further both in relation to other UK and international studies.

Some of these inequalities appear even starker, when international comparisons are made. *Greater Expectations* indicates that if the UK was doing as well for children as the best industrialised nations:

- almost one million children in the UK would not be living in poverty;
- 172 fewer children would die each year, due to unintentional injury;
- At least 300,000 more 15–19-year-olds would be in education or training;
- 770,400 fewer children under 15 would be living in poor environmental conditions.

(3)

We will be returning to some of these statistics, as we move in turn to health, poverty and education. Clearly, no 12 indices can be comprehensive, but they provide a backcloth to further analysis within the chapter.

The health of UK children

The health of UK children is probably one area where statistics are both reasonably comprehensive and have been collected over a sustained period. At the beginning of the chapter, reference was made to the RCPCH's 2017 assessment of child health in the UK, with the muted assertion that we could do better. After all and incontrovertibly: "A vital and productive society with a prosperous and sustainable future is built on a foundation of healthy child development" (4, p. 5).

Just as there was an acknowledgement, in Chapter 1, of the huge strides that had been made in improving the lives of children in the last 50 years, so too any consideration of areas where children's health in the UK is still poor, needs to be tempered by positive assertions about the progress that has been made. So, at the beginning of the twentieth century one in six infants did not live until their first birthday in the UK (infant mortality rates were around 150 to 160 per 1,000 live births). Today, infant mortality is 3.9% per 1,000, meaning that only one in 256 infants do not reach their first birthday. Equal gains in general health have been seen not only across childhood but also adolescence. Nevertheless, as the 2017 RCPCH asserts, inequality still "blights our children's lives" (1, p. 6) and comparatively, as we shall see, the UK does not emerge high in some international health and well-being league tables.

Infant and childhood deaths provide a useful touchstone for the overall health of children and young people. Infant mortality can be divided into neonatal mortality – deaths up to 27 days after live births – and post-neonatal mortality – deaths from 28 days but under one year. The percentage of babies born weighing less than 2,500 grams ranged from 3.4% to 9.8% in most European countries. Here, preterm birth rates in the UK were higher than in the Nordic countries and lower than in Germany, Spain and Belgium (5). At the same time, the UK appears to have the highest still birth rates of a sample of 12 comparable high income countries. Every year, an estimated 1,951 additional children (around five a day) die in the UK compared with Sweden – Europe's best performing country for child mortality. Some 60% of the UK's child mortality takes place in the first four weeks and is often the result of babies being born prematurely (6). Similarly, death rates from illness that rely heavily on "first access" services (for example, meningococcal disease, pneumonia and asthma) are higher in the UK than in Sweden, France, Italy, Germany and the Netherlands (7).

Lastly, before turning from infant death to other aspects of child health, the NHS Atlas of Variation in Health for Children and Young People (8) reveals significant regional variations in perinatal mortality in the UK (comprising all stillbirths and babies born alive but who die within seven days of birth). This is largely attributable to health and social risk factors, such as obesity, smoking, ethnic background and rates of teenage pregnancy. That there should be such variation points to the inconsistency with which health is delivered across regions.

While some aspects of childhood present difficulties for the statistician, keen to demonstrate whether children's health and social well-being is improving or declining, this is not the case for some aspects of health. It is quite the opposite: where we have a richness of data across, for example, disability, obesity and diabetes, non-intentional injury, teenage suicide and mental illness. An inevitable starting point, which becomes particularly important when we look at regional variations, is the connection between poverty, inequality and poor health. In an influential review of health inequalities Marmot found that "there is a social gradient in health – the lower a person's social position the worse his or her health" (9, p. 3). In parenthesis, the social inequalities affecting children in the original *Born to Fail?* report, considered above, were still having a significant impact on children's well-being in the follow-up report. Marmot continues by arguing that disadvantage accumulates throughout life and that there is a close link between early disadvantage and poor outcomes over time. An example, quoted by Marmot, is that people on low incomes often refrain from purchasing goods and services that can improve or maintain health, perhaps because they cannot afford them. They may also feel that they have no alternative but to buy cheaper goods and services that can, in turn, increase health risks. All of this, of course, strengthens the argument for the need to ensure that services for children embrace all aspect of their lives.

One of the first markers of childhood good health is to be found in breastfeeding rates. Two statistics stand out here: first, the minimal progress in breastfeeding rates since data collection commenced and, second, unfavourable comparisons with some other European countries. If the medical benefits of breastfeeding are accepted, we find only 44% of mothers were recorded as breastfeeding at their six to eight week health visitor review in 2014–15 and this represents little improvement on 2009–11 figures (1). As the RCPCH report also concluded: "An analysis of global breastfeeding prevalence at six months found that in the UK only 34% of babies are receiving some breastmilk, with 49% in the US and 71% in Norway" (1, p. 32).

Needless to say, and following on from Marmot, a 2010 infant feeding survey demonstrated that 46% of mothers in the most deprived areas were breastfeeding, compared with 65% in the least deprived areas.

In terms of comparisons, the UK has some of the highest rates of teenage pregnancy (10) with teenage levels highest amongst young women in the most deprived areas (1). And if this is linked to the issue of smoking in pregnancy, given that smoking is one of the most important modifiable risk factors for improving health, it remains the case that England and Scotland's rates of smoking during pregnancy in the UK are higher than in many comparable European countries.

Media reporting of child health statistics have increasingly focused on the twin headline grabbing issues of obesity (and the accompanying medical complications of diabetes) and adolescent mental health. Obesity is one of the initial 12 indicators in the original NCB study (2) and tracked in the NCB follow-up (3). The Chief Medical Officer's 2012 report on children's health concluded that "currently 12.5% of toddlers are obese, 17% of boys and 16% of girls up to the age of 15 are obese too" (11, n.p.). A central message, both from the NCB report (3) and RCPCH (1) is the strong relationship between deprivation and overweight/obesity prevalence. Furthermore the 2013 NCB report recorded that "boys living in deprived areas are three times more likely to be obese than boys growing up in affluent areas and girls are twice as likely" (3, p. 24). Similarly, the RCPCH report (1) concluded that, in England, it appears that overweight and obesity amongst children may be reducing over time in the least deprived but not amongst the most deprived. Those seeking a cause for the rise need look no further than the UK consumption of sugary soft drinks, compared with some other European countries, such as Finland and Sweden (3), and the diminishing amounts of time being spent by children in exercise and outdoor pursuits.

Linked to the growth of obesity is the rise in Type 2 diabetes. This is normally associated with adults but, as a childhood condition, is affecting a growing number of children and young people in the UK. Not only does the NHS Atlas of Variation in Healthcare (8) reveal significant demographic differences between deprived and well off areas in the UK, but those from deprived or black and minority ethnic backgrounds have higher risks of the disease.

If we accept the evidence of a link between an increase in sugary drinks amongst children and obesity, it is not surprising that tooth decay is also a significant public health issue for children. Despite tooth decay being almost entirely preventable, 31% to 41% of five-year-old children across the UK have evidence of tooth decay, with rates higher for those in deprived populations (1). As a result, tooth decay – and tooth extraction – is the most common single reason why children, aged five to nine require admission to hospital.

Two childhood conditions also requiring attention because of wide geographical variations and unfavourable comparisons with some other parts of Europe, are asthma and epilepsy. In terms of the former, the UK has one of the highest prevalence, emergency admissions and death rates for childhood asthma in Europe. There are also wide variations in the incidence of asthma across England, which the RCPCH speculates may reflect improvements in care in the best performing health authorities, rather than deterioration in the worst (8). One *British Medical Journal* report records that about 75% of all children's asthma admissions could have been prevented with better primary care. Furthermore, in the context of the wider thesis of this book, over a third of short-stay admissions to hospital in infants are for minor illnesses that could have been managed in the community (7).

Turning to epilepsy, this is common in childhood, affecting approximately 48,000 children in England. Again, there are wide geographical variations, with the greatest prevalence in deprived populations (8). In examining some of the regional variations, RCPCH has concluded that the greater availability of community-based support, such as specialist epilepsy nursing services, could well contribute to reducing some of these regional variations.

Another common indicator across both NCB surveys relates to absence rates from school, due to illness. If absences for medical or dental appointments are excluded, there is evidence to indicate that children receiving free school meals have more absence than those who do not. Although this statistic needs treating with caution, we might speculate that this is further evidence for the link between greater levels of deprivation and poorer health.

A further indicator of child health inequality can be found by comparing accident rates. The Black Report not only identified accidents as one of the most important causes of death among children (between 1 and 14 years) but also one of the causes of childhood mortality with what the report called the "steepest socioeconomic gradient" (12). In other words, the risk of accidental death for all children between 28 days and 15 years was considerably higher amongst unemployed people than for a child with at least one parent in a higher managerial or professional occupation, a finding confirmed by the NCB study (3). On a smaller scale this conclusion is also borne out by an article in the *British Medical Journal*, which looked at Tower Hamlets, as one of the most deprived inner-city London boroughs, and demonstrated a positive correlation between injury rates by home address and income deprivation. In other words, the most socioeconomically deprived children are at greatest risk of injury (13).

Before moving on from children and health, there are some issues that surround the teenage years, namely alcohol, drugs, suicide and mental illness. Drugs were not a significant issue to be recorded in the original NCB report and, equally, alcohol use was not included. However, in the RCPCH report (1) alcohol and drugs – specifically cannabis use among young people – while significantly declining over the last decade still mean that the UK ranks poorly amongst other European countries. England, Wales and Scotland are ranked 16th, 21st and 22nd respectively out of 42 European countries that reported 15-year-olds drinking alcohol at least once a week.

When we come to examine both suicide and mental illness in young people, there is a strong association between growing up in deprivation and risk of suicide or mental illness. A recent study of suicide deaths from 2001 to 2011 found that in England the mean rate of suicide among 15–19-year-olds living in the most deprived areas was 79% higher than for those living in the least deprived areas (1). Similarly, when we examine mental illness, children in the poorest households are three times more likely to have a mental illness than children in the "best off" households (14) with the BMA concluding that a greater reluctance to access services amongst deprived groups may result in mental health issues becoming more severe before assessment and support can be provided.

Finally, in this section, a UNICEF report into the wider issues of child well-being looked at 29 of the world's more advanced economies. They were ranked in terms of overall well-being, material well-being, health and safety, education, behaviour and risks, housing and the environment. These 29 countries included America, Canada and a range of European countries. Overall, the UK was placed 16 out of the 29 (being particularly low in terms of education – 24 out of 29) and 16 for health and safety. Education is self-explanatory, but it is important to note that health and safety included infant mortality rates, low birth rates and child deaths (15).

So what can we conclude about UK healthcare for children? Three factors emerge strongly. First, the link between low income and deprivation and poorer levels of health in children; whether this is measured against teenage suicide rates, low birth rates or obesity, for example. Second, as the NHS Atlas of Variation indicates, that there are other wide variations between English regions as a result of differing levels of affluence and the relative performance of health authorities.

Third, and this will be explored more fully in the book, that one of the reasons why the UK appears to perform worse than other European competitors, in terms of health, is the way in which health services for children are organised. "A better balance is needed between accessibility and expertise for first access and planned care for children" (7, p. 903). In the same article Wolfe et al. explain models in other European countries where the co-location of services appears to lead to better outcomes. To avoid the challenges of many different appointments with a multitude of professionals "teams should comprise jointly trained general practitioners and paediatricians working with children's nurses, health visitors, allied professionals and mental health professionals" (7, p. 903) all located in the same place. A message we will hear repeated.

Children and poverty

Turning now to childhood and levels of poverty in the UK, we are first faced with two definitions. While there are numerous ways in which poverty can be measured, usually it is evaluated in one of two ways – in relation to a defined level of income know as *relative* poverty or in relation to a defined amount of income needed to meet basic needs (known as *absolute* poverty). Relative measures of poverty compare the income of households with the average income in a country. Within the UK this is set at 60% of the current median (or middle) income. But even this is complicated, since it can be expressed before housing costs or after (i.e. including) housing costs. Absolute measures of poverty use a fixed threshold that only rises with inflation and represents a certain level of income needed for basic goods and services.

Poverty amongst children figures in two of the National Children's Bureau's indicators and in both of the reports. Indicator 1 looked at the number of children living in poverty and indicator 2 at the proportion of children living in poverty by family circumstances. In the original report (2), the NCB calculated 2 million children living in poverty, which had risen to 3.5million in 2013 (3). But, as the NCB notes, while this represents a substantial increase, it is difficult to make a direct comparison due to changing definitions. These figures are based on the Institute for Fiscal Studies, which has recorded poverty rates since 1961. The NCB further asserts that the figures will rise further – by more than one million by 2020 – with a then estimated 4.7 million children living in poverty.

In the 2017 RCPCH report (1) nearly one in five children in the UK was calculated as living in poverty; a figure again predicted to increase (6). This is based on relative poverty figures with income less than 60% of the median (16). For the RCPCH the logical link is between poverty and ill health, but the implications are far wider. A *Save the Children* report (17) tracked how poverty permeates all aspects of family life: having to hold back on food, going without shoes or clothes, missing out on educational opportunities (see below) and increasing levels of unhappiness or stress. One report puts the costs of child poverty at around £25 billion a year, through a combination of extra spending by government and lost taxes (18). The Save the Children report graphically records the direct experience of families for whom poverty is a very real and daily issue.

Children and education

The further link, often made, between poverty and early years care, also helps to make the transition to educational achievement for children in the UK. A report from the Joseph Rowntree Foundation (19) on the impact of high-quality early education and effective early intervention, indicated that those in poverty were often the poorest users of such services. First, because families in areas of low parental employment are less likely to have access to flexible child care and, second, because support with child care costs does not work well for low income parents. The message from the report is a call for an anti-poverty child care system that both maximises and removes the barriers of affordability and access to parents on low incomes.

Education is an area where international comparisons are difficult because of the very varied systems in place. In terms of the UK, however, the NCB's follow-up study (3) has four indicators relating to education: namely the number of children in early education; the proportion of four-year-olds who achieved a "good level of development" in the Early Years Foundation stage; the proportion of 11-year-old pupils achieving the expected level in English and Maths and the proportion of 16-year-olds achieving five or more A–C grade GCSEs excluding English and Maths. In terms of early years education the vast majority (96% of 3 to 4-year-olds in England) attend some early education (93% of 3-year-olds and 98% of 4-year-olds).

There has been a significant increase in the proportion of children receiving early education, since *Born to Fail?*, although those from poorer backgrounds were less likely to achieve "a good level of development" in the Early Years Foundation stage. If eligibility for free school meals is taken as a yardstick, 64% of all four-year-olds achieve "a good level of development" during their early years education, while only about half (48%) of children on free school meals achieve this level.

In terms of the school years and, again, almost five decades on from the original NCB survey, there is little indication of the gap between advantaged and disadvantaged children at school disappearing. Today, a child from a disadvantaged, poorer background is still more likely to achieve a lower academic level than peers. This gap continues at GCSE level, with far fewer disadvantaged pupils achieving at least five A–C grade GCSEs, including English and Maths.

In *Born to Fail?* the NCB found that growing up in disadvantage understandably had a negative impact on children's educational outcomes and on the expectation of continuing in learning beyond the age of 16. Almost 50 years on, the inequalities remain. A quarter of children from poor backgrounds fail to meet the expected attainment level at the end of primary school, compared with 3% from affluent backgrounds.

This gap widens at 16, with only one in five children from the poorest families achieving five good GCSEs, including English and Maths, compared with three quarters from the richest families.

While it is the case that international education comparisons for children are difficult, the UNICEF report into child well-being (15) does take education as a comparator amongst the 29 countries surveyed. According to the classification, indicators of education included, first, participation rates in early childhood education and also in further education (15–19-year-olds), second, the percentage of 15–19-year-olds not in education and employment or training and, third, scores across reading, maths and science, as measured by the PISA (Programme for International Student Assessment Rates). While educational well-being was seen to be the highest in Belgium, Finland, Germany and the Netherlands, the United Kingdom was 24th amongst the 29 countries.

Two elements of the UK's poor educational performance are particularly noticeable: first, the not unsurprising variation in achievement between those from deprived and better off families and, second, the wide variety in regional results. The second of these is particularly noticeable because regional patterns have changed in the last few years.

In the 2017 Social Mobility Commission report (20) there is an unequivocal statement that there remains an unbroken correlation between social class and educational success. In England, as a whole, only 39.2% of pupils on free school meals achieve A to C grades in English and Maths GCSE, with 67% for all other pupils. These findings are borne out by a report from the Centre for Social Justice (21) warning that children from the poorest homes risk becoming an "educational underclass", starting school nearly two years developmentally behind their peers. As the report points out, falling behind at the very beginning of school can be the starting point for permanent disadvantages.

The second issue, one of regional variations, is made both by the Social Mobility Commission and an earlier Ofsted report (22). The conclusion from both reports is that the national distribution of underachievement has shifted in recent years. Twenty or 30 years ago the problems were in the big cities. So, inner London schools might have been the best funded but were the worst achieving in the country. Now, schools in inner and outer London are the best performing and achievement in other big cities, such as Birmingham, Greater Manchester, Liverpool and Leicester has also improved. Instead, where the most disadvantaged children are being let down by the education system is no longer deprived inner city areas. Instead, the focus has shifted to deprived coastal towns and rural, less populous regions of the country, particularly down the East and South East coast of England. These are places that have felt little impact from national initiatives designed to drive up standards for the poorest children.

Flesh is further put on this argument by the Social Mobility Commission. They describe "hot" and "cold" spots where educational achievement is largely good or bad. So, disadvantaged children are 14% less likely to be reading when they enter school at age five in cold spots than in the hot spots:

- In Kensington and Chelsea 50% of disadvantaged youngsters make it to university.
- In Hastings, Barnsley and Eastbourne university participation rates for this group is just 10%.
- In England as a whole only 39.2% of pupils on free school meals achieve A to C in England and Maths GCSE, compared with 67% for all other pupils.
- In cold spots, disadvantaged young people are almost twice as likely to be not in education, employment or training after GCSEs, half as likely to gain two or more A levels and half as likely to enter higher education that those in hot spots *(20)*

Variations, between regions, both in terms of the level of services and corresponding educational achievement, provide further evidence of the need for joined up, integrated services.

The protection of children

The protection of children from abuse, whether emotional, physical or sexual is one area where national interest is high but data collection difficult. First, because, as stated earlier, the data itself does not always go back over a long period of time, permitting rigorous analysis and, second, because in terms of international comparisons, countries tend to record child protection statistics in different ways. Again, we need to preface a consideration of data associated with child protection with an acknowledgement that, in some ways, children are safer from abuse and neglect today than those of previous generations. However, evidence from the NSPCC indicates that in recent years there has been an increase in recordings of emotional abuse, as a reason for children being on a child protection plan. In 2016/17 there was an increase in the public reporting of child abuse, an increase in police recorded child sexual offences and indecent image offences across the UK and more children on child protection plans. Furthermore, knife crime has grown, with the number of teenagers and young adults stabbed to death in England reaching the highest level for eight years, with a total of 215 for the 12 months up to March 2017. The Crime Survey for England and Wales, reporting on the year ending in December 2017, recorded a 22% increase in offences, involving knives or other sharp instruments.

Returning to the NSPCC report, and equally concerning is that "More than one child a week dies because of maltreatment . . . and one in five children today have experienced serious physical abuse, sexual abuse or severe physical or emotional neglect".

A useful indicator, used by the NSPCC, is the number of children subject to a child protection plan (CPP) or on the Child Protection Register (CPR). Evidence reveals that between 2004 and 2015 the number of children in the child protection system increased in all four nations: the greatest increase took place in England, where the rate increased from 24 to 43 per 10,000 (1). This particular measure only includes children who have been identified as at risk of or are experiencing harm and, therefore, is unlikely to capture the true number of children who are at risk. We need also to recognise that thresholds for evaluating risk can alter between local authorities and a greater awareness of child protection issues – often the result of tragic child deaths – can lead to fresh initiatives to lower the thresholds to register "at risk" children. (See below for more information of social care thresholds.) In England and Wales neglect and emotional abuse are the most common primary reasons for children being on a CPP or CPR. Neglect, physical and multiple abuse were the most common categories in Northern Ireland and, in Scotland, emotional abuse, neglect, parental substance misuse and domestic abuse were the most common causes (1).

While the death of a single abused child in the UK is wholly unacceptable, the NSPCC statement that one child a week dies through maltreatment is a sad indictment of a country that boasts the fourth largest economy in the world. And, as the NSPCC points out, new kinds of threats are emerging; particularly with the increasing amount of time children spend in the digital world. As many as one in four 11–12-year-olds experience something on a social network site that concerns them almost every day (23). It is also likely that the on-line world will figure much more largely in future child protection data.

The significance of this data is that children who experience physical or emotional harm can continue to live with the effects into adulthood (1). These can be reflected in emotional difficulties, mental health issues, drug or alcohol misuse, poor physical health or lower educational attainment. All of this data becomes important when we begin to examine which models of care might help to alleviate the effects of childhood abuse.

Two final points deserve making and take us back to the NHS Atlas of Variation in Healthcare for Children. First, are the regional discrepancies for those who end up in care and, second, lower achievement levels for those in the care system itself. With regards to the first of these, a 2016 National Audit Office report (24) concluded that not only is the quality of help and protection for children both unsatisfactory and inconsistent, but that children in different parts of the country do not get the same access to help or protection. The report found that there was a lack of a common understanding or application of thresholds- the level of concern at which child protection enquiries are triggered. In some cases, thresholds were being set too high or too low, meaning that some children were not being referred to social care or being referred inappropriately. In the financial year ending 31 March 2015 there was variation between local authorities in the rates of:

- referrals acted upon from 226 to 1,863 per 10,000 children; and
- children in need from 291 to 1,501 per 10,000.

In addition, children living in deprived areas are 11 times more likely to have a child protection plan than children living in the most affluent areas of England. In regional towns, what this means is that a child in Blackpool is nearly eight times more likely to be in local authority care than one in Wokingham, Berkshire. Similarly, a child in Wakefield is almost nine times more likely to be referred to social services than one little more than 30 miles away in York.

These figures are particularly significant, because children who experience the care system often have poorer life chances and achievements than other children. We have already explored educational achievement levels between those from deprived and poor backgrounds in comparison with the rest of the young population. For those in care, the outcomes are even worse.

Looked-after children

In a chapter on statistical data, associated with UK children, it is clearly important to give consideration to those specific children whom the state has removed from their carers. Children subject to a care or placement order, living in foster or residential care, provide a distinct group within the wider population of UK children. For many such children, care provides a positive experience, opening up opportunities that might otherwise not have been presented. But in terms of educational achievement and overall well-being, the cohort of looked-after children have poorer outcomes than children not in the care system. Now, of course, this could be the result of early life events, their subsequent experience of care or a combination of the two.

If we take education, for example, at Key Stage 1, attainment for both looked-after children and children in need is much lower than for the rest of the population. (Only 37% reached the standard for writing, compared with 66% in non-looked-after children (25).) The same is broadly true at Key Stage 2 and at Key Stage 4. If we look at exclusions from school, the rate of permanent exclusions for looked-after children is around twice as high as the rate for all children. Looked-after children are more than five times more likely to have a fixed period of exclusion than all children.

Similar results were found in Scotland, where looked-after children tended to leave school at younger ages and with lower/fewer qualifications than all school leavers (26). This study also discovered a correlation between the number of placements a child had and subsequent qualifications: often the more placements, the lower the qualifications.

Looking more widely at outcomes for looked-after children, Doug Simkiss examined a group of health issues affecting adults who had previously been looked-after children. He concluded that they were less likely to attain high economic status, more likely to be homeless, more likely to have psychological problems and more likely to be in poor general health than those children not brought up in care (27). For those who experienced multiple placements, they sometimes missed out on health checks, with incomplete immunisations and increased evidence of, for example, dental caries and asthma. There is also evidence to suggest that they are more likely to experience mental illness than their peers. All of this is particularly important when we consider that children are often removed because the state deems they are not properly protected by existing carers. Failure to redress the effects of early deprivation provides another dimension in our questioning of current services for the most disadvantaged children in our society.

Conclusions

While Chapter 3 explored the way we fail children, with governments launching a stream of short-term initiatives, each replaced by more fresh ideas, this chapter looks at the kind of quantitative data that makes comparisons and conclusions possible. That the National Children's Bureau should repeat a survey of children from poor, disadvantaged backgrounds, almost 50 years after the first, provides a unique opportunity to measure progress. The conclusion that "poverty and inequality experienced by our children remain just a prevalent today as it did 50 years ago", led the NCB to a number of questions as to whether we want every child to have the same life chances, regardless of their parents' means and whether as one of the richest nations on earth we shouldn't have greater expectations for children in the UK.

In terms of progress and in a similar way, the RCPCH repeated the 2017 *State of Child Health* report in 2018 (28). The report found the state of child health "largely unchanged". Child poverty was it its highest level since 2010. One in three 11-year-olds were overweight or obese and 100 out of every 1,000 young people under 19 are likely to have a diagnosable mental health disorder.

The figures, relating specifically to increased levels of child poverty, are supported by 2018 statistics from the End Child Poverty Coalition (29). Devising a new child poverty map of the UK, broken down by parliamentary constituencies, the Coalition concluded that there are now constituencies within the UK where more than half of children are growing up in poverty, compared to one in ten, in the areas with the lowest child poverty rates.

What we might conclude is that while poverty and certainly obesity in childhood is increasing, we also have higher rates of teenage pregnancy than some other European countries and more infant deaths. Furthermore, that poorer children achieve less educationally and that the effects of disadvantage find their way into poorer health and educational outcomes. Evidence, both from the NHS Atlas of Variation (8) and the work of the Social Mobility Commission (20), indicates that there are often significant variations in levels of service and therefore outcomes, in differing parts of the UK. Education provides a particularly vivid example of this with poor educational performance shifting in recent years from inner city areas, like London and elsewhere, to rural and sometimes coastal areas where performance is now often poorer.

While international comparisons are often difficult, the UNICEF report (15) which places the UK 24th out of 29 according to a series of "well-being" indicators, strongly suggests we have some distance still to travel. As the RCPCH report (1) concludes, inequality still "blights children's lives in the UK" and leads to the inevitable question as to whether services are being delivered in the best way. It also leads on to questions about value for money and cost effectiveness, which Chapter 5 will explore further.

Notes

1 *State of child health*. Report, no author, 2017, Royal College of Paediatrics and Child Health, London.
2 *Born to fail?* The National Children's Bureau reports on striking differences in the lives of British children. Wedge, P. and Prosser, H., 1973, Arrow Books in association with the National Children's Bureau, London.
3 *Greater expectations. Raising aspirations for our children*. National Children's Bureau, 2013, London.
4 *The foundations of lifelong health are built in early childhood*. Center for the Developing Child, 2010, Harvard University, National Scientific Council on the Developing Child.
5 *Why children die: deaths in infants, children and young people in the UK*. Wolfe, I., Macfarlane, A., Donkin, A., Marmot, M. and Viner, R., 2014, RCPCH, NCB and British Association for Child and Adolescent Public Health, London.
6 *We can stop children dying if we change*. Attwood, K., 2015, *The Independent on Sunday*, 8 March.
7 *How can we improve child health services?* Wolfe, I. et al. 2011, *British Medical Journal*, 23 April, vol 342, 901–904.
8 *NHS atlas of variation in healthcare for children and young people*. NHS, March 2012, London.
9 *Fair society, healthy lives: the Marmot review*. Strategic review of health inequalities in England post 2010. 2010, University College, London.
10 *Getting it right for children and young people: overcoming cultural barriers in the NHS, so as to meet their needs*. Kennedy, Sir Ian, 2010, Department of Health and Social Care, London.
11 *Prevention pays: our children deserve better*. Chief Medical Officer, 2012, Press Release, Thursday 24 October.
12 *Inequalities in health – report of a research working group*. Black, D., Morris, J., Smith, C. and Townsend, P., 1980, Department of Health and Social Security, London.
13 *Childhood injury in Tower Hamlets one of the most deprived inner-city London boroughs: prospective audit date from the Royal London Hospital*. Kourita, L., Jameson, J.D., Kirkwood, G., Smith, D. and Pollock, A., 2013, BMJ, November 29.
14 *Growing up in the UK. Ensuring a healthy future for our children*. BMA Board of Science, 2013, British Medical Association.
15 *Child well being in rich countries. A comparative overview*. UNICEF, Innocenti Report Card 11, 2013.
16 See also *Living standards, poverty and inequality in the UK: 2015–16 to 2020–21*. Browne, J. and Hood, A., 2016, IFS Report R114, Economic and Social Research Council.
17 *Child poverty in 2012. It shouldn't happen here*. Whitham, G., 2012, Save the Children Fund, London.
18 *Estimating the cost of child poverty*. Hirsch, D., 2008, Joseph Rowntree Foundation, York.
19 *Creating an anti-poverty childcare system*. Butler, A. and Rutter, J., 2016, Joseph Rowntree, York.
20 *State of the nation*. Social Mobility in Great Britain, 2017, Social Mobility Commission.
21 *Requires improvements. The causes of educational failure*. The Centre for Social Justice, September 2013, London.
22 *Unseen children: access and achievement 20 years on. Evidence report*, Ofsted report, 2013, Ofsted, Dorset.
23 *How safe are our children? The most comprehensive overview of child protection in the UK*. Bentley, H., Burrows, A., Clarke, L., Gillgan, A., Glen, J., Hafizi, M., Letendrie, F., Miller, O., O'Hagan, O., Patel, P., Peppiate, J., Stanley, K., Starr, E., Vasco, N. and Walker, J., 2017, NSPCC, London.

24 *Children in need of help or protection*. National Audit Office, Department for Education, October 2016.
25 *Outcomes for children looked after by local authorities in England*. Department for Education, 31 March, 2016, London.
26 *Looked after children: education outcomes 2015–16*, Scottish government, June 2017.
27 Outcomes for looked after children and young people. Simkiss, D., 2012, *Paediatrics and Child Health*, September, vol 22, issue 9, 388–392.
28 *State of child health: one year on*. Royal College of Paediatrics and Child Health, January 2018, London.
29 *More than half of children now living in poverty in some parts of the UK. Improving the lives of children and families*. End Child Poverty coalition, 2018, Press Release, 24 January.

5

THE COSTS OF CARING FOR CHILDREN

How can we cost child care?

So what is it we spend, looking after children in the UK? Trying to arrive at a figure that encompasses not only health and social care but also education, leisure and the voluntary sector (and this excludes, for example, libraries, employment schemes for young people and welfare benefits) is a daunting task. It is like medieval maps of the world, where the known continents are tentatively delineated but beyond was boldly written "there be dragons". The dragons in this case are fed by failures either to break down and separate adult and children's services or to reach a consensus on what has actually been spent. Furthermore, unless you remain especially vigilant, double counting some of the expenditure is all too easy. A good example of the latter would be health and social care allocations, which first appear in the government's overall spending budget but then become distributed to individual health and local authorities.

If further evidence of the challenges we face were needed, the UK government's response to Article 4 of the United Nation's Convention on the Rights of the child (which puts an onus on states to establish a children's budget), provides a warning: "Identifying the proportion of Government spending which is allocated to children is difficult for a number of reasons" (1).

It continues by outlining what these are. First, the UK government has a policy of devolving budgets to the front line. Second, at a national level, some funding supports all age groups and is not disaggregated solely for children and young people. Third, it is often difficult to ascertain how government support, paid to families, is used for the individual benefit of children within the household. If it is true that governments find it difficult to ascertain how much they spend on children, then this difficulty will be replicated all the way throughout the system.

Despite this government "health warning" about allocating expenditure, there have been a number of calls to calculate what it really costs to look after children. In a report from Save the Children, in 2009, the charity called both for transparency in how resources are directed to children and a leavening out of the differences in costs to deliver the same services in various parts of the UK:

> Investment in children needs to be visible, accountable and transparent. Establishing children's budgets at a national and local level will enable greater understanding of and greater transparency around public spending on children.
> *(2, p. 2)*

The problems of discussing these costs are legion as we, first, attempt to compartmentalise costs, second, fail to budget for the costs of not providing services and, third, argue that specific areas like health are underfunded. Each of these deserves some consideration.

Calculating the unit cost of a young man sent to prison is a good example of compartmentalising costs. To assert confidently that it costs, on average, about £35,000 a year to keep someone in prison (3) says little about the overall costs that have accumulated over the years before this incarceration. Given that a considerable percentage of those in adult custodial settings were looked-after children, with periods in care, they may well have experienced foster homes or residential care, extra educational and psychological support and police involvement – all of which will have incurred considerable costs. The problem is that no one, as the Americans say, "does the math" in order to arrive at a total figure. It is highly probable that the total cost of caring for the young man up to and including his prison sentence would be well beyond that of, say, a public school education. However, no one department has overall responsibility for measuring or controlling the accumulated costs, which is probably why we never address the fundamental question as to whether this could be managed better or if the state is really getting value for money.

But the problems go further. On the one hand we have no global figure for providing care for children but, conversely, we have little idea of the costs associated with not doing so. The Marmot review into health inequalities not only examined the shorter life spans of those living in the poorest neighbourhoods but the knock on costs of not investing and consequently allowing health inequalities to flourish. Marmot estimated that the annual cost of health inequalities is between £36 billion and £40 billion, through lost tax, welfare payments and costs to the NHS (4). Poverty, he argues, can lead to ill health and the subsequent additional demands on NHS and other services. As far back as 2009 the Save the Children Fund was arguing that "not ending child poverty has high costs for our society. It has been estimated that child poverty costs the UK at least £35 billion per year" (2, p. 5). Even at a micro level, the Centre for Mental Health estimated that the long-term consequences of failing to address severe behavioural problems, which often start in children, could result in lifetime costs of £260,000 per individual (5). They are twice as likely to leave school with no qualifications, six times more likely to die before 30 and 20 times more likely to end up in prison. The other side of this coin – equally difficult to calculate – is the belief that investment in education, increasing opportunities by widening choice for young people or policies such as tax credits, aimed at reducing poverty, will increase life chances and, consequently, decrease the costs to state services.

Because we have little idea of the global costs of caring for children, arguments often focus on the specific amounts that individual departments spend. Health is a good example of this. Writing specifically and now historically of the NHS in 2010, Professor Sir Ian Kennedy stated that:

> The total allocation to the NHS is around £10 billion. The overall amount spent on children and young people is not clear (which may itself say something) but DH (i.e. the Department of Health) estimates that the figure is around £6.7 billion. The RCPCH offers the estimate of £3.1 billion (2007). The Healthcare Commission put the figure at £3.2 billion (2008).
>
> *(6, p. 28)*

We will later return to this global health figure, when we examine the NHS budget in more detail. The NHS Atlas of Variation takes the discussion on, arguing that whatever the true figure is, there are considerable savings to be found in this (disputed) global figure:

> Total NHS spending on children's healthcare services has been estimated at £6.7 billion. Reducing unwarranted variation in healthcare by eliminating inefficiencies can save commissioning bodies millions of pounds, through the redeployment of resources.
>
> *(7, p. 11)*

Health is used here as an exemplar of the wider problems. Not only will we struggle with a global figure of what is spent on children's services, but also with the individual parts of the whole, like health or social care. And, of course, not having certainty about what is spent makes it more difficult to argue whether or not it is either well allocated or sufficient

Government spending on children

The logical starting point has to be the UK Government's annual budget, which determines the overall amounts to be spent on their principal areas of responsibility. For 2018/19 the total estimate for public sector expenditure was calculated to be around £809 billion. Of this, the largest allocation went to social protection or policies to reduce poverty and vulnerability, caused by unemployment, exclusion, sickness and disability. Health is the next largest, accounting for £155 billion, or 19% of the total budget, followed by education (12%) or £102 billion. Personal Social Services accounts for 4% of the total budget or £32 billion (8). What makes these figures a challenge, in terms of working out how much of this can be allocated to children's care, is that health, education and personal social services and also social protection encompass both adult and children's services.

One of the few attempts to disaggregate these figures on a smaller but albeit national scale, was initiated by the Dartington Social Research Unit in Northern Ireland. They devised a method of "fund mapping" (9), which broke down the budget across the 12 government departments that had some responsibility for children. As the report warns however, "the preparation of a children's budget is a surprisingly complex task. There is not, as yet, an acceptable methodology" (p. 20).

Northern Ireland's total public expenditure for 2012/13 was just over £15 billion, of which £2.28 billion was spent on services for children, young people and their families. The highest spending ministry was education with £1.89 billion of the total children's budget, followed by health, social services and public health and then employment and learning.

From a total population in Northern Ireland of 1.8 million people, with 432,000 aged under 18 (or 24% of the total population), it was possible to calculate that £5,175 was spent annually in Northern Ireland on every child and young person. Yet – and this illustrates the challenge of determining global figures – it excludes the population-wide spend on, for example, infrastructure, GPs or other primary care costs or emergency services.

If we look at the way in which the report broke down education, subdividing the spend in terms of preschool, primary and post primary education, the authors conclude that the biggest allocation is, not surprisingly, on post-primary education. Northern Ireland has also made a significant investment in youth services, special schools and Sure Start projects and the report also examines this as part of the overall allocation. There was also a considerable voluntary sector contribution to Northern Ireland's children's services made by the children's charity Barnardo's and which will be examined further in Chapter 6

What the Dartington study reveals is, first, that we don't yet have the metrics for determining accurate data for overall costs of services to children. As the authors conclude, while there is reasonable data on what was spent, it is not possible to be as clear about how it is spent in any detail. Second, that we need to devise ways of choosing whether this spend goes towards prevention, mainstream services or the targeting of those in greatest need.

What the remainder of this chapter will explore is conclusions we can draw about the way this global expenditure for the UK government is divided across health, social care, education and leisure using the public information that is available. The voluntary and private sectors will be considered separately in Chapter 6.

Health costs

Four major themes dominate any consideration of health spending in the UK:

- the distribution of health costs, based on age;
- the challenge – again – of disaggregating adult from child health costs;
- the allocation of health costs, specifically to preventive care;
- the unit costs of services.

If we begin with health spending linked to age we find, not surprisingly, that costs grow exponentially with age. More than two-fifths of national health spending in the UK is devoted to people over 65. An 85-year-old man costs the NHS about seven times more, on average, than a man in his late 30s. Costs rise steeply over the age of 50, with people over 85 costing an average of £7,000 a year. In terms of children, the comparatively high costs incurred around birth and up to the age of one quickly diminish and health spending on childhood per se remains low in comparison with the older groups of the population.

But disaggregating costs between adult and children's services remains very tricky. Treasury data reveals that, in real terms, spending has more than doubled for health from 1994 to the present day. Health is the service for which public expenditure has increased the most in the last 20 years. As a proportion of gross domestic product, this represents an increase from 5.2% to 7.3% in the same period (10). But with a growing elderly population a large part of the debates about health spending are, for the above reasons, centred on providing for this over 65 population. This is also reflected in discussion about integration of health and social care for elderly services.

The challenge of allocating costs in health is that clinical staff, such as anaesthetists and surgeons, may well work across children and adult services. So, attributing costs to, say, children's pathology or radiology services is very difficult. Similarly, if we examine primary care, about 25% of GPs' caseloads are in paediatrics but again are not separately accounted for (11). Added to this complication is the extra cost of services like children's hospices, which are largely voluntary funded and don't therefore appear on any NHS balance sheet.

If we return to the Dartington research work on children's child care costs in Northern Ireland, their research revealed that the joint Health and Social Care Boards spent £479.9 million on children and young people, with £292.5 million on health and £187.4 on social care. Of the health allocation the biggest share was on obstetrics, paediatrics, child and adolescent mental health and health visiting, with the rest going towards areas including midwifery, school nursing and psychology services. To be able to replicate this division of expenditure across the whole of the UK would be useful in terms of comparing costs.

What we do have, however, is some work completed by Kent University on what they describe as "reference costs" for selected children's health services (12).

Their calculations take account of the direct costs of clinical staff, indirect costs, such as laundry and lighting, and overheads associated with running the organisation. So, to provide examples, the net average cost of a speech therapy session is £98, an outpatient consultation with a paediatrician £261 and £252 for a visit to a mental health specialist team. These are little more than indicative costs, but, as we shall later see, the same interrogation of social services costs, again undertaken by Kent University, is useful at identifying a much wider range of community based interventions.

Lastly, in relation to health costs, it is sometimes stated that in the UK there is a national sickness, rather than health service. Responsibility for developing preventive health strategies lies largely with public health and is now within the remit of local government. Over recent years, governments have cut the grant it gives to local government for public health (13). In 2015/16 local authorities also took on public health responsibilities for 0–5 year children's services. Again, it is difficult to separate public health spending on children from that of adults. However, even allowing for the temporary boost in funding, when local authorities took over responsibility for the 0–5-year-olds, the King's Fund indicates a year-on-year reduction in public health spending (a fall of 5.2% between 2013/14 to 2017/18). This has taken place when the UK is faced with a growing public health problem of obesity amongst children and young people, more sedentary lifestyles and a growth in child and adolescent mental health. All of these are areas where preventive public health policies can make a difference and reduce costs further down the line.

Social care

Allocating how much local authorities spend on children's services is slightly easier than determining health costs. Typically, councils budget to spend nearly twice as much on adult care as on children – largely a reflection of the growing elderly population. The National Audit Office (NAO) has calculated that of the 152 English local authorities, £16.8 billion was ring fenced for adult social care, in 2016/17 and £8.6 billion on children's social care (14). Interestingly, the NAO also calculated that £108 billion of informal, unpaid, care is further provided by families and carers. Of course, this will be a combination of care to both adults and children, but it again illustrates the difficulty of reaching an overall global figure of the amount spent on children.

That this overall figure is not adequate to provide council services for children has been argued by the Local Government Association, who calculated that, in 2015/16, 75% of councils exceeded their children's social care budgets by a total of £605 million. Furthermore, that, unless this were addressed, the figure would reach an overspend of £2 billion by 2020 (15).

If we break down the overall total of £8.6 billion then of the three largest categories, £1.9 billion was spent by local authorities in relation to the 621,470 referrals for children in need requiring help or protection. A further £2.6 billion was used to support 70,440 looked-after children and £282 million to help those leaving the care system.

In relation to the first of these categories – children in need of help and protection – there has been an exponential rise in the number of referrals for help in recent years. The Local Government Association has published figures indicating that the number of children subject to child protection enquiries has increased by 151% in 10 years, from 73,800 in 2006/7 to 185,450 in 2016/17 (16). These figures are largely confirmed by the NAO, which reported a 94% rise in the rate of children beginning child protection plans in a ten-year period leading up to 2015 (17). This is usually attributed to the number of child protection enquiries, following tragic deaths, such as Victoria Climbié, Daniel Pelka and Peter Connelly; all creating a climate within which local authorities have not been seen to intervene to protect children early enough.

This increase in child protection work has also been accompanied by wide regional variations, both in terms of the number of children helped and the money allocated. Again, the NAO estimated that in 2014–15 the average spending ranged from around £340 per child in need, in one authority, to £4,970 per child in another. More concerning, the report concluded that there was no relationship between spending per child in need and the quality of service offered by the local authority (14).

If we then turn to the average costs of looked-after children, we again find wide regional variations. Costs between 2015/16 for looked-after children varied between £52,000 for the highest and £39,000 for the lowest, with an average of just over £45,000 (18). Similarly, rates for children in need varied in 2015–16 between just over £8,000 per child and £12,750 in the highest spending authorities.

Lastly, in relation to local authority spending on children, the Personal Social Services Research Unit (12) have been able to produce useful unit costs in more detail than was available for health. The fact that children's services are more easily separated from adult social care makes a significant difference in allocating costs. So, for illustrative purposes, if we choose a few examples, we learn that the cost of keeping a child in a local authority children's home was, on average, £3,860 per residential week at 2016 prices. Foster care, by comparison, costs £634 per child per week and the cost of an adoption is, on average, £27,000, whether this is through a local authority or a voluntary adoption agency. Post-adoption support, in addition, is on average £7,845 – including health, social care, education and financial support. The cost of short breaks in residential accommodation varies between £80 and £463 per night, depending on the degree of disability and Local Children's Safeguarding Boards (which have a responsibility to coordinate agencies involved in child protection) cost, on average, £169,000 a year to run. These are, to some extent, random examples, but if we were able to achieve the same degree of granularity in terms of what individual services cost, then we could not only reach an overall figure but begin to make meaningful comparisons between regions and districts.

What all of the above figures exclude is a combination of costs that parents and carers need to find for child care together with the central government contributions through tax relief and the benefits system. In terms of the former, the Family and Childcare Trust (FACT) estimated that parents or carers of primary school age children pay, on average, £53 a week for an after school club or £67 for the pickup and aftercare by a childminder (19). Child care costs families about £6,000 a year, or about £116 a week for the expense of a part-time nursery place for a child under two. In 2017 the government introduced tax-free child care for some families across the UK and a roll-out of an increased entitlement to 30 hours per week of free child care for working parents of three- to four-year-olds in England. FACT estimated that as a result of these changes £7.2 billion of public funding, which constituted 0.48% of GDP, would be allocated to child care spending. In terms of that elusive global figure of what we spend on children, this is clearly a significant sum.

Education costs

Again, education spend is slightly easier to calculate than that of health. We saw, earlier, that for 2017/18, the overall government's estimate for public sector expenditure for education was £102 billion, about 4.4% of the GDP, and the next largest element of public service spending in the UK, after health. Government spending on education grew by about 1.7% per year in real terms over the 1980s and 1990s, before increasing sharply during the 2000s by more than 5%, in real terms (20). With the exception of education spent on 16–18-year-olds, most education has been protected from cuts since 2010–11. Since education is a devolved matter, it is funded separately in the other UK nations and these figures relate solely to England.

Chancellors periodically provide a 4/5 year view of the government's overall spending plan, to indicate future directions. The 2015 spending plan for education envisaged investing over £1 billion more a year by 2019–20 in free child care places for two- to four-year-olds, £23 billion capital investment over the period of the parliament to open 500 free schools, provide over 600,000 additional school places, rebuild and refurbish over 500 schools and address essential maintenance needs of schools. From 2019–20, the government also intended to spend a record £6 billion a year supporting parents with their child care costs, including tax-free child care and Universal Credit. The enormity of these global figures helps to establish the financial context within which education operates (21).

Not only can we gain reasonably accurate figures for the total current spending on education in England, but we can break this down into early years, schools, further education and sixth form.

Early years is one area where spending has grown exponentially. As recently as the 1990s, early years spending was less than £100 million a year at 2016–17 prices. By 2015/16 this had risen to about £2.3 billion. If we include within these costs the entitlement to 15 hours of free early education for three- to four-year-olds, Sure Start projects, tax free employer child care vouchers and subsidies through Working Tax Credit, then the figure is almost £5.4 billion (2016–17 prices) (20).

If we turn to schools, the spending per pupil is about £4,900 in primary school and £6,300 at secondary level. The Institute for Fiscal Studies estimates that spending per pupil has almost doubled in real terms between 1997–8 and 2015–16 as a result of successive governments prioritising school spending. Overall, total spending on schools in England was £39 billion (2016–17 prices) in 2015–16 or 11.5% of total public service spending in England (20).

Turning, finally, to further education and sixth forms, the total spending on 16–18 education in England was about £6 billion in 2015/16. If we break this down, £2.2 billion went to school sixth forms and £3.7 billion was allocated to further education and sixth form colleges (20).

What this consideration excludes, is a raft of other education costs, ranging from academy schools to sport in schools and – once again – the contributions from the purses of parents and carers. In 2017 the Northern Ireland Commission for Children and Young People estimated that parents spent more than £1,200 per child each year (22) on things like uniforms and school meals

Equally excluded from our consideration are those who either home school or are educated within the independent sector, where costs can be over £18,000 a year for an independent day school or £30,000 a year for a boarding school. The Good Schools Guide 2017 calculated that educating a child who starts boarding school aged seven may have cost half a million pounds in fees, by the time s/he reached 18 – the equivalent to that of a small castle, as the report points out! Similarly, the growth of the academy schools movement, discussed in Chapter 2, often involves additional financial support from personal or corporate sponsors. Also to be included in this evaluation is the increasingly large percentage of parents or carers who supplement their children's education with private tutors. And, lastly, the Office for National Statistics estimates that, after transport, recreation and culture alongside housing are the largest source of expenditure for families and children (23). Part of this will be both for sport and arts activities for children, which parents finance either as part of or additional to what is offered by the schools. This list of additional expenditure is by no means comprehensive, but helps to illustrate, once again, how challenging it is to arrive at global figures for what we spend on children.

No consideration of children's services' funding would be complete without examining the contribution of the voluntary sector nor of the private sector. Today, again, the voluntary sector is collectively adding a large contribution to the overall spending on children. It fact, it is so significant that Chapter 6 will explore this aspect separately, alongside that of private providers. This is for two reasons. First, because of the net contribution to the overall budget spent on children but also because the scale of their involvement is such that they deserve special consideration in any discussion about an integrated child care system. Any attempt to aggregate the total amount being devoted to the care of children cannot afford to ignore the contribution of private and voluntary sector providers.

So what can we conclude?

First, that we have not – by any means – exhausted the balance sheet of income dedicated to children's services in the UK. Take, for example, the monies allocated to libraries, leisure services and playgrounds. Understandably, none of these figure largely on the pie charts of central government spending and are largely the responsibility of local authorities. In the case of leisure centres and playgrounds, however, there has also been a significant input of national lottery sports funding, in recent years. In 2016/17 what is broadly defined as culture and leisure amounted to £2.2 billion, but this would, of course also include adult services (14). It is an area where cuts in local authority services have been particularly severe, with what the same report records as a reduction of 34.7% between 2011–12 and 2016–17.

One-off allocations have helped; with the Department of Culture, Media and Sport, as it then was, providing evidence that, in the year to April 2016, 21,218 schools had participated in the School Games project, with £17.9 million of public funds being allocated. This was part of a competition, first established in 2011, for school-aged children between the ages of 7 and 19 and aimed at increasing the pool of young people eventually able to compete in Olympic and para-Olympic games (24).

In terms of library and leisure services it is, once more, impossible to disaggregate what percentage of these are allocated to children, as opposed to adults. Libraries and leisure services have also been easy targets for stretched local authorities having to find additional savings to put into adult social care.

We have seen earlier that debates about the levels of funding going into caring for children are confined to specific services and not to the global sum spent on children. Where debate about the current size of the overall social care budget for children has taken place it has generally been about early years' services. An argument that has widespread acceptance amongst the major political parties has been that investing in nurseries and early years provision helps to move the focus towards a preventive, rather than a reactive service. We can see this reflected in Sure Start and Family Centre projects, tax and Child Care Credits and the expansion of early years' provision, referenced earlier in this chapter.

Taking the debate about the cost of prevention further, was a report by Action for Children and the New Economics Foundation *Backing the Future: why investing in children is good for us all* (25). The argument that the rewards of a preventive approach are both economic as well as social, led the report to look at what we might save by delivering services differently.

The central thesis of *Backing the Future* is that children's services are built on a model of "curing" rather than fixing the underlying problems – the same argument we have heard earlier in relation to an NHS "illness" as opposed to a "health" service. The report argues that the costs of the UK's social problems far outstrip those experienced by other European countries. If indicators such as obesity, crime, those not in employment or training, mental health problems and child abuse are taken into account, the comparative costs of dealing with these social problems is higher in the UK than a sample of 15 other European countries.

The report further argues that to do nothing to improve social problems in the UK, over the next 20 years will cost £3 trillion. Taking the indicators of obesity, crime etc. outlined above and putting in extra resources would involve an additional spend of £620 billion over 20 years. This roughly means doubling current

GDP expenditure on children and families from 2005 levels of 3.2% to 7% by 2030. However, as the report concludes: "Even with our conservative estimates, the combined investments in targeted and universal services would together provide net savings of £880 billion" (p. 7). To complete the report's arguments, it is proposed that this is financed by bonds, issued over a ten-year period.

The report is considered here because it illustrates the challenges and issues we face. The argument, in terms of greater investment for long-term preventive reasons, will now be familiar to readers. But the calculations based on a series of social and health problems that currently exist take little account of what the future may throw up. Furthermore, the report makes no attempt to reach a global figure spent on children's services, which earlier parts of this chapter have also tried to address. From time to time, the argument is raised that we should divert a large percentage of money spent on child protection investigations, for example, into preventive services. But the courage needed to do this, in the face of public scrutiny of child abuse, has always eluded politicians and local councils.

We have little choice but to conclude that, in the UK, we do not know with any accuracy what we are collectively spending on children. If we take recent debates about the charitable sector, for example, and which we will explore further in Chapter 6, it is tempting to ask if there is not duplication or whether taking out the infrastructure costs of similar organisations wouldn't allow for some rationalisation. It is equally tempting to ask if, at a gross level, we may, indeed, have enough to spend on a first class system of care for children if it were distributed in different ways. But difficulty in arriving at the overall figure makes this conclusion tricky.

What we can conclude with more certainty is that a more integrated system, which linked up health, education, social care, leisure and the voluntary sector, for example, would permit a more accurate investigation of costs and the potential to reduce waste and duplication where it does occur. This will be the major focus of Chapter 8.

Notes

1 *Consideration of reports submitted by states parties under Article 44 of the Convention. United Kingdom.* UN Convention on the Rights of the Child, 2015.
2 *A child's portion. An analysis of public expenditure on children in the UK.* Sefton, T., 2009, Save the Children, London.
3 *Annual report and accounts 2016–17.* National Offender Management Service, 2017, HM Government, London.
4 *Fairer society, healthy lives.* (The Marmot review) Marmot, M., 2010, Institute of Health Equity.
5 *Building a better future: the lifetime costs of childhood behavioural problems and the benefits of early intervention.* Parsonage, M., Khan, L. and Saunders, A., 2014, Centre for Mental Health.
6 *Getting it right for children and young people: overcoming cultural barriers in the NHS so as to meet their needs.* Kennedy, Professor Sir Ian, 2010, Department of Health and Social Care.
7 *NHS atlas of variation in healthcare for children and young people.* 2012, NHS.
8 *Autumn budget 2017.* HM Treasury, November 2017.
9 *Fund mapping: the investment of public resources in the wellbeing of children and young people in Northern Ireland.* Kemp, F, Ohlson, C., Raja, A., Morpeth, L. and Axford, N., 2015, Dartington Social Research Unit, NICCY, Belfast.

10 Data produced for *The Guardian*, 1 February 2016.
11 I am indebted to Dr Hilary Cass, former president of the Royal College of Paediatrics and Child Health.
12 *Unit costs of health and social care 2017*. Curtis, L. and Burns, A., 2017, Personal Social Services Research Unit, The University of Kent, Canterbury.
13 *Local government spending on public health: death by a thousand cuts*. Buck, D., 2018, The Kings Fund, London.
14 *A short guide to local authorities*. National Audit Office, October 2017, National Audit Office.
15 *Child services face £2 billion gap over funding*. Weale, S., *The Guardian*, 9 August 2017.
16 *Bright futures. Children's services facts and figures*. Local Government Association, 2017, London.
17 *Children in need of help or protection*. National Audit Office, October 2016, London.
18 *Children's services: spending and delivery*. Department for Education, 2016, researched by Aldaba and the Early Intervention Foundation.
19 *Childcare Survey 2017*, Harding, C., Wheaton, B. and Butler, A., Family and Childcare Trust, 2017.
20 *Long-run comparisons of spending per pupil across different stages of education*. Belfield, C., Crawford, C. and Sibieta, L., 2017, Institute for Fiscal Studies, London. I am grateful to the Institute for Fiscal Studies for figures in this section of the chapter.
21 *Department for Education's settlement at the spending review 2015*. Press Release, Department for Education, 25 November 2015.
22 *The cost of education for families in Northern Ireland 2016–17*, 2017, Northern Ireland Commissioner for Children and Young People, Belfast.
23 *Family spending in the UK: financial year ending 2017*. 2018, Office for National Statistics.
24 *School games indicator 2015/16*. 2016, Department for Digital, Culture, Media and Sport, London.
25 *Backing the future: why investing in children is good for us all*. Action for Children and the New Economic Foundation, 2009, New Economics Foundation, London.

6

CARING FOR CHILDREN IN THE VOLUNTARY AND PRIVATE SECTORS

Several years ago I visited a children's centre in the middle of a large, deprived northern city. It was bustling with prams, children and notices for activities, ranging from yoga to a breastfeeding clinic, keep fit and antenatal classes. I asked the officer in charge if she had a list of other voluntary organisations for children and families in the two inner city districts that fed into the centre's catchment area. As if she had anticipated the question she produced a large piece of paper that looked like the wiring diagram of Concorde. On it she had charted the range of voluntary organisations that, through individual projects, were offering services to children and their families. There were literacy and language classes, delivered by a local voluntary organisation but funded by the local authority and targeted at the large Asian population that had settled in the area during the last 20 years. There was a specific service for the Romany travellers, again municipally funded but organised by another local charity. There were three nurseries, one specifically aimed at families with a disabled child, again voluntary funded; five playgroups; an after school club; a project for mothers experiencing post-natal depression; and a housing advice centre. The list was considerable, including hostels and drop-in centres, often focused on specific health, social welfare, advice and financial support and in some cases deliberately targeting specific parts of what was a very mixed community. Some projects were funded by local authority grants, some from central government funding, three or four large voluntary organisations were contracted to run services by the city and the remainder provided by voluntary organisations from their own funds.

When I asked the manager about coordination and cooperation she was both measured and pessimistic. There were pockets of cooperation and examples of organisations that did work together, but it was easier to find examples of non-communication and duplication. The example was given of two literacy schemes, both aimed at the same parts of the community but funded from different sources and existing independently of each other. The local council of voluntary services kept a reasonably current register of voluntary child care organisations, but did not have a role in bringing organisations together to avoid duplication.

Margot Jeffreys reached similar conclusions as far back as 1965 in a survey she did of social welfare provision in the county of Buckinghamshire (1). Even then, and this included adult as well as child care services, there was the NSPCC, a missioner for the deaf, an old people's welfare service, the Citizens Advice Bureau, a worker from what was then the National Spastics Society (now Scope) and at least half a dozen other agencies. While this is far from an objective, scientific or wide-scale survey, this example and the experience of the children's centre manager go some way to questioning whether whether integration between various parts of the voluntary child care sector has still not been achieved.

The origins of charities

The history of voluntary sector child care is a good illustration of the way in which some wheels really do come full circle. The Charitable Uses Act of 1601 established four purposes for charitable activities:

1. The relief of poverty;
2. The advancement of education;
3. The advancement of religion; and
4. Other purposes beneficial to the community.

The same year, the Poor Relief Act instructed parishes to accept responsibility for destitute children. It was as a result of these two pieces of legislation that voluntary organisations became established and grew in power and influence, reaching a peak in the nineteenth and early twentieth centuries. While State provision was largely confined to the operation of the Poor Law, charities began establishing themselves to fill gaps in provision. For example, Lewis, in tracing the role of the former Charity Organisation Society (which became the Family Welfare Association) from its roots in 1869, states that, as recently as three years before the onset of the First World War, the gross annual receipt of registered charities exceeded all public expenditure on the Poor Law (2).

Organisations like Dr Barnardo's Homes, the National Children's Home (which eventually became Action for Children) and the Waifs and Strays Societies (later transformed into the Church of England Children's Society) owe their origins and growth to the nineteenth century. At the time of its founder's death in 1905, Barnardo's was looking after 11,277 children (3), eventually spreading the work to countries like Australia, New Zealand and Ireland. Similarly, men like Thomas Stephenson and Lord Shaftesbury were founding charities that continued long after their deaths.

A good example of this was the Thomas Coram Foundation, established even earlier, in 1739, with the intention of providing for children abandoned on the streets of London. Its eponymous founder established the Foundling Hospital, in the face of, at best, public apathy and, at worse, a callous disregard for human life (4). It was partly based on the Ospedale degli Innocenti for foundlings in Venice where the composer Vivaldi was a supporter. Mothers were permitted to leave their children at a door in the hospital, knowing that the child would be brought up for a life in service (girls) or the armed forces (boys). This, understandably, pre-empted one of the most fiercely fought and still contemporary debates in the delivery of social welfare. By offering help in this way, were you condoning vice and, indeed, encouraging its continuance? Many of the children would have been illegitimate and would now be provided with a living, or were you simply and pragmatically responding to a need that if left unanswered would lead to misery and death?

What we have seen in Chapter 2 is that the whole raft of change, during and following the Second World War led to the State becoming the principal source of provision for children, across health, education and social care. As a result, the voluntary sector began to decline. Children's homes, for example, were now largely run by the state and as children's departments gave way to generic Seebohm social services departments, the voluntary sector was left providing a more peripheral role in support for children. The NSPCC dropped its position as "the cruelty man", investigating child protection, with the state now assuming these statutory responsibilities. Up until the onset of the first Margaret Thatcher government in 1979, there was a consensus that education, health, public utilities, the criminal justice system and the civil service, were public services. However, this was to change again as many of these services were opened up to new providers. With the State contracting its services – in both senses of the word – the landscape was about to change yet again.

So, the 1980s and 1990s saw a dramatic change to public services. As Jones records:

> The changes relate to changes in power, control, funding and responsibilities and have redefined the "market place" (indeed even the terminology!) in which we understand the role of the state and public services. While the power, control, funding and responsibilities for public authorities may all be seen to have changed (usually by being reduced), the focus on consumer choice and on performance and value for money has increased.
>
> *(5, p. 40)*

Jones defines five major ways that resulted in this sea change. First, ways of funding were altered to make it easier for money to be – again – directed towards voluntary organisations (and, as we shall later see, the private sector). Second, regulation and regulatory bodies were changed, to make this possible. Third, there was some agreement that a few residual bodies could remain with public sector agencies, such as child protection, but much else could be run by other bodies. Fourth, there was a whole new set of ways for reporting on performance, such as school league tables and patient waiting lists, to measure how new providers were performing. Lastly, the government argued that this greater range of providers was a direct response to demands for more consumer choice and a greater say in how services were run. As a result, the relationship between the state and voluntary organisations for children became more complex, both in terms of the scope of the relationship and also with regards to the rules and processes that determine this relationship (6). As we saw in Chapter 2, the same new level of complexity also affected the NHS, largely as a result of the Lansley proposals and the subsequent Health and Social Care Act 2012.

We shall shortly see that this new range of opportunities or threats – depending upon your political viewpoint – also affected private providers of care for children. What is significant, here, in terms of arguments about integrated child care, is that it has led to a new continuum, which, at the one end, has voluntary sector services that are directly commissioned and entirely paid for by local authorities or, in fewer cases, central government funding and, at the other, voluntary sector child care services that rely entirely upon charitable funds raised in the traditional ways.

We shall look at the funding of the larger children's charities below. Sufficient to say here that some of the big voluntary sector providers are now running services such as fostering and adoption, supporting young carers, after care support, juvenile justice, child sexual exploitation and leaving care services. In some cases they have had to compete against each other or private sector providers for local authority contracts. And even smaller independent voluntary organisations in towns and cities bid to run specific services. Grants have given way to more formal contracts.

The development of private sector child care

This cannot claim to have the long history that the voluntary sector possesses. But again, the recent growth in private sector child care was precipitated by the Thatcher governments. The National Health Service and Community Care Act 1990 not only created a right for people to have services tailored to their individual needs but introduced what became known as the "internal market". Basically, the state became an "enabler" rather than necessarily a supplier of health and social care provision. Local authorities continued to assess the needs of the local population and then purchased the necessary services from "providers". To become providers, health authorities became trusts, competing, as it were, with each other to win contracts. As a consequence, by 2016, 66% of children's residential homes were run by private sector and private equity firms; 47% of foster care and 14% of social work was provided through independent, largely profit-making companies with companies like G4S, Serco and Virgin Care bidding for new work (6).

In Devon, for example, Virgin Care won the contract in 2012 to provide what was described as an integrated children's service on behalf of Devon County Council and the North, East and West Devon Clinical Commissioning Group.

Effectively, Virgin Care were commissioned to provide, among other areas, specialist school nurses, an autism spectrum assessment service, child and adolescent mental health services, children's nursing, family support and a learning disability team. The CAMHS service alone generates 33,500 appointments a year for children and young people with mental health issues.

The NHS Support Federation has calculated that over 60% of NHS contracts are now won by non-NHS bodies. The cost of this market is difficult to calculate but estimates vary between £4.5 billion and £10 billion a year (7). The report also estimates that the number of contracts awarded to the private sector since the Health and Social Care Act has increased sevenfold. These range from ambulance services to out of hours support, services for older people, community and hospital services.

Opening up services to the private sector has aroused considerable controversy, particularly within the health and social care professions. Of particular concern was the possibility that child protection services might also be tendered to private sector providers who would be able to conduct child protection investigations and assessments. In 2014 the Department for Education set up an innovation programme, looking at the delivery of services and this was followed by proposals that although the private sector should not be free to run sensitive services, like child protection, they could set up not for profit subsidiaries, to run the services and charge the management and administration costs back to the main provider.

These developments are important in that they illustrate how complex the current funding and range of provision for children is today. While it is possible to gain some broad figure of the amount the voluntary sector contributes to the global budget for delivering children's services, and we will look at this below, it is impossible to know how much is being contributed by the private sector itself. Of course, at one level this is not new money but money the private sector is being awarded to run services previously provided by, say, local and health authorities. We have no idea how much money the private sector is providing itself; either as "seed money" or to take on "unprofitable" services on the basis that it provides a foot in the door with, say, a local authority. "Lost leaders" as other aspects of the private sector would describe it. But two things are vital for the arguments in this book. First, that both private and voluntary sector provision for children is here to stay. Second, that when we come to outline an integrated service we need to be mindful that private and voluntary sectors will want to play a significant part.

What the voluntary sector contributes to children's services

In estimating the voluntary sector's financial contribution to the overall children's services' budget we might start with what the general public contribute. Children and young people remain one of the most popular causes. The CAF report, on public donations to charities revealed that in 2017 £10.3 billion was donated to charities in the UK (an increase from the 2016 figure of £9.7 billion) (8).

During a four-week period surveyed, children and young people were the third most popular cause for donations (23%) after medical research (26%) and animal welfare (24%). In 2017, the overall proportion of total donations received by each cause was 19% to religious organisations, 19% to animal welfare and 7% to children and young people. According to the National Council for Voluntary Organisations, there are 65,368 charities devoted to children. Overall, in 2013–14 they raised £6.1 billion in voluntary income – that is, money raised from the general public (9). Of course, this includes a huge cross section from organisations like Great Ormond Street (which raised £92 million in 2016–17, according to their annual report), Mencap, the Cystic Fibrosis Trust, children's hospices and the Guides Association, for example, to small charities such as parent teacher associations and playgroups.

If we return to the Dartington research into income for child care services in Northern Ireland (Chapter 5), it looked at the contribution made by the charity Barnardo's (10) to the overall funding. At the time of the survey, Barnardo's had 45 services in Northern Ireland and, out of a total expenditure of £13.5 million, £10 million of this came from the statutory sector; money that was obtained by undertaking work on behalf of the Northern Ireland Health and Social Care boards. In other words, the bulk of the income received by Barnardo's in Northern Ireland did not come from fundraising and shaking buckets outside shops but from directly contracted work for which, in some cases, they would have needed to compete.

This pattern is true of Barnardo's across the UK. In 2016–17 Barnardo's – running more than 1,000 services and reaching 240,000 children and young people – achieved income of over £301 million. Of this, £172.6 million was from statutory income or the money received from local authorities to operate many of those services that councils would previously have run. Evidence from the annual reports of some of the other major voluntary providers of children's services, indicates a similar pattern:

With the NSPCC, the number of children helped is more difficult to calculate or compare. The overall figure includes children reached through, for example, school assemblies. With the exception of ChildLine, the charity has largely moved away from providing direct services and into campaigning and research work on behalf of children and young people. If we were to include Save the Children in the survey (although their remit is not just to work in the UK but internationally),

TABLE 6.1 The amount of statutory income received by Action for Children, the NSPCC and The Children's Society 2016–17 (11)

Name of charity	*Number of children helped*	*Total income (£million)*	*Statutory income (£million)*
Action for Children	370,000	159.8	135.5
NSPCC	1,802,500	127.4	12.7
The Children's Society	13,000	41.6	7.051

it dwarfs all of the other children's charities with an overall income of £1,072 billion in 2018 (12). In parenthesis, we might also note that voluntary income from Barnardo's, Action for Children, NSPCC and The Children's Society (i.e. money they raised themselves from the public) exceeded £431 million in 2016–17, a substantial addition to the overall amount going into caring for children.

How does the voluntary and private sector fit in?

As we have seen, the voluntary and private sectors operate differently when it comes to directly contracted work. In the case of the private sector, they are often taking over areas of work previously performed by local or health authorities. This may also be the case with the larger voluntary organisations, like Barnardo's or Action for Children, but there are also thousands of small voluntary sector providers, running playgroups or groups for children with disabilities. Sometimes they are financed with funds raised from local contributions and sometimes with grants from the host local authority in which they work. For some, they are run on a wing and a prayer, never sure of permanent funding and always hopeful that, like Mr Micawber, some (statutory) income will turn up.

Large voluntary organisations sometimes make a contribution from their own funds, to secure a contract. This might be because it gives the charity a competitive edge or because the offered service fits in with an overall mission. Barnardo's, for example, as part of their overall strategy, have provided a series of challenging services in the area of child sexual exploitation, where voluntary funding has helped to supplement some services run directly on behalf of local authorities.

In an analysis of this new relationship between voluntary sector and state, Jones (5) goes further in describing at least four examples of new collaborations between state and the voluntary sector:

- There is the purchaser relationship, outlined above, where state agencies purchase services directly from voluntary organisations.
- There are competitive relationships where the state might find itself competing with the voluntary sector for business.
- Collaborative relationships where state and voluntary sector work together.
- Advocacy relationships, where the role of the voluntary sector is one of advocate or pressure group on behalf of a specific group of children and young people.

Few areas of child care have invited so much controversy as the engagement of the private sector in previously state-run services. For supporters of this new landscape, the private sector has brought a new commercial edge to the way services are delivered, some reduction in overall costs in certain cases and the development of new models of child care that can be rolled out in different parts of the country. They see the private sector as being more focused on outcomes (because of the nature of the contracts) and better at evaluating how much services cost.

For opponents of private care, recent developments have meant costs have been cut to the detriment of quality and what is not in a contract does not get done. It is inevitable that in contracting services, so the argument goes, commissioners will be looking to find those who can run the service cheaper than they could themselves. Statutory organisations, like health and social services, have been forced to learn commissioning skills, which are traditionally more familiar to private sector colleagues. If an area of practice is omitted from a contract there may be the need to add extra clauses to include the new work and invariably this will push prices up. And while private providers are subject to external inspection, it may be more difficult to establish the same inter-agency links that develop when services are run "in house", as it were, by health or local authorities.

With regards to the voluntary sector, the pros and cons are slightly different. Positively, they bring their own funding, which can be used to boost services or they use their own strategic priorities to feed into those of local authorities. But a more fundamental concern of voluntary sector services takes us back to the "Concorde diagram" that began this chapter. By developing services in a locality (particularly those that are wholly or substantially funded from voluntary income), there may be an absence of joining them up with other services. The decision to place a children's centre, for example, in a deprived community can always be justified on the basis that it will inevitably help to fill some social needs. But it may contribute to the wider dispersing of services that are not fully joined up and result in a series of uncoordinated or duplicated facilities. And those who are contracted to provide services sometimes complain that they have little influence in contributing strategically to the way that the overall needs of a defined population of children and young people might be comprehensively met.

The commissioning of services from voluntary or private sector providers is vital to later arguments about an integrated model. Both the voluntary and private sector are here to stay. But in devising an integrated model, we need to find a better way of making sure that both voluntary and private providers are absolutely focused on the totality of children's care in a locality and not just an adjunct to it.

Notes

1 *An anatomy of social welfare services: a survey of social welfare staff and their clients in the county of Buckinghamshire.* Jeffreys, M., 1965, Live Issue Series, Michael Joseph, London.
2 Quoted in *Sweet Charity: The role and workings of voluntary organisations.* Hanvey, C. and Philpot, T. (Eds) 1996, Routledge.
3 *Champions for children, the lives of modern child care pioneers.* Holman, B., 2001, The Policy Press, Bristol.
4 *Thomas Coram, Gent.* Wagner, G., 2004, Boydell Press, Woodbridge.
5 Jones, R. Swimming together: statutory and voluntary in *Sweet Charity* (see 2 above).
6 New report is the next step to privatising children's social services. Jones, R., 2016, *The Guardian*, 12 December.
7 *Contracts failures. Failed contracts reveal cracks in the NHS market model.* NHS Support Federation, 2018, Brighton.

8 *CAF UK giving 2018: overview of charitable giving in the UK.* CAF UK, 2018, West Malling, Kent.
9 *Financial analysis of the children and young people's voluntary sector in England.* NCVO Civil Society Almanac, 2017, London.
10 *Fund mapping: the investment of public resources in the wellbeing of children and young people in Northern Ireland.* Kemp, F., Ohlson, C., Rajan, A., Morpeth, L. and Axford, N., 2015, Dartington Social Research Unit, Dartington.
11 Information provided from the 2016–17 Annual Reports of Barnardo's, the Children's Society, Action for Children and the NSPCC.
12 *UK's Top 10 Children's Charities by Income revealed.* Charity Financials, Wilmington, 2018.

7

THE CASE FOR INTEGRATION

"Integration" has become an "aerosol" term that can be liberally sprayed but is rarely or properly defined. If we are to escape Lewis Carroll's Humpty Dumpty who petulantly asserted that "when I use a word it means just what I chose it to mean" we need to strive for a more meaningful and shared working definition.

When integration is spoken about, in the context of public services, it usually focuses on conveying a coming together of health and social care departments. However, not only is common usage confined to the joining of health and social care but it is more often than not meant to imply only adult or, more specifically, elderly services. To a large extent, this narrow definition has been precipitated, in the UK, by the growing crisis of supporting an ageing population. With elderly people living longer, being admitted to hospital and then eventually requiring additional support on their discharge back into the community, public services have struggled to meet this demand. Unless health and social care departments work closely together, beds become blocked and those providing community support or domiciliary services are not able to keep up with the growing demands made. Hence the call for greater integration. In January 2018 the Secretary of State for Health extended his ministerial portfolio by taking on responsibility for social care; partly a response to the growing crisis facing hospital and social care for the elderly.

This is not to say that other aspects of adult services have not looked at the issue of integration. For example, the MEAM (Making Every Adult Matter) (1) initiative focused on those with multiple needs facing homelessness, substance misuse, criminal justice issues and mental ill health. They have been assisted by a coming together of community safety services, the police, health, alcohol nurses, housing, the ambulance services, local landlords and mental health specialists, in an initiative largely led by the voluntary sector.

When we turn to children's services the focus is somewhat different. Calls for integration have been more nuanced, mainly because of a combination of the wide range of agencies that impinge on children's lives and the many differing ranges of support that children need. Earlier, in Chapter 3, we explored a number of national initiatives that, in different ways, attempted to achieve some degree of integration for children. These included the Troubled Families programme, Children and Adolescent Mental Health services and Extended Schools. They all represented very different efforts to bring together various service providers at differing periods in children's lives, such as mental health, addressing educational inequality or early years. In this chapter we will examine more local and sometimes individual attempts at bringing services together, including overseas examples, in order to learn from them and to define some principles of successful integration. There will also be a consideration of how integration has been played out in some other countries.

Integrating social care

Over the last few years there has been no shortage of rhetoric or slogans to indicate that joining up care for children is a desirable outcome. Two of these – "wraparound child care" and "the team around the child" – are more honoured in the breach than the observance.

Wraparound child care originated in the early 1980s, originally as a means of helping young people with serious emotional problems in their homes and local communities. It aimed at a network of friends, family and agencies coming together to provide support and has a resonance with the African proverb that it takes a village to raise a child – made popular by Hillary Clinton's book, published in 1996 (2).

In the UK, the Department for Education gave wraparound child care a more narrow definition, referring to that child care that schools provided outside of normal school hours, such as breakfast clubs or after school activities.

"The team around the child" (3) was popularised by the Children's Workforce Development Council and linked to the idea of a lead professional who would bring together the people closely involved in a whole intervention system for the child and family. This lead professional would be the first point of contact, coordinating the delivery of services.

We shall see, later in the chapter, a number of significant arguments for joined up or integrated health services and the same arguments have been made in relation to social care. In 2014 the Local Government Association published a consultation document, outlining their ambition for children and young people (4). It stated that what people want more than anything is for services to be built and integrated around the needs of children and their families: the key principle underpinning these proposals was the need for decision-making for public services to be brought together in one place, with this "re-wiring", as they described it, taking place around the needs of the users - children and families.

Sometimes, the calls for greater integration for children's services have been made in relation to specific groups of children. So, for example, in 2017 the Lenehan review examined the support that was needed for children with multiple needs.

This focused specifically on the 2.5% of the general population with a learning disability: 40% of whom will also experience significant psychiatric disorders (5). The report argued for "wraparound support" – that phrase again – which aimed for "good multi-agency approaches". In order to ensure the provision of better services for children, the report called for a clear joint agency commitment at the highest level with shared access to the service, its costs and funding. What is also implied here is a new model of funding that permits budgets to be pooled in some way. An argument to which we will return in Chapter 8.

Similar arguments for integration, affecting a comparable group of children, were reached by the Family Fund. The Fund provides individual grants for low-income families with disabled children and looked specifically at the issue of sleep deprivation experienced by many of their carers. "Tired All the Time" (6) examined a sample of over 2,000 parents and carers raising disabled children. Over 93% were awake in the night with their children and approximately half experienced health issues, due to sleep deprivation. As a consequence, they had consulted paediatricians, neurologists, GPs, social workers and health visitors and usually faced a lack of any coordinated approach. For the Family Fund this was an inter-professional issue, requiring sleep services that brought together health, education and social care.

Lastly, in terms of calls for the integration of services and in relation to specific groups of children, the charity 4Children called for a new model of child and family centres for vulnerable families experiencing drug or alcohol dependency, mental health problems or domestic violence (7). It was argued that they could become multipurpose "hubs" for local families and their communities. Such centres would bring together and coordinate services ranging from midwives and health visitors to child care, out of school and youth support. Again, the idea of a child care "hub" is one to which we will return in Chapter 8.

Examples also exist of where integration has been tried, albeit on a small scale and not necessarily with the same groups of children. These experiments have taken place in areas as diverse as North Yorkshire, Hackney, Newcastle and Surrey. The list is by no means exhaustive, but they serve to show how very varied populations have addressed some degree of social care integration for children.

"No Wrong Door" was developed in North Yorkshire, specifically to work with young people who were within or on the edge of the care system. It replaced traditional council-run young people's homes with hubs that combined some residential care with foster care provision. Two initial hubs – one in Scarborough and the other in Harrogate – had a dedicated team consisting of a psychologist, speech therapist, two community foster families and community-supported lodgings. A Department of Education report on the scheme in 2017 (8) looked at the 355 12- to 25-year-old young people who had been supported between 2015 and 2017. Working with other agencies in this way indicated there had been success in keeping them out of the care system, decreasing the number of placement moves, helping programme their education and training, reducing offending and helping with the transition to independent living.

Arising from the 2011 London riots, the borough of Hackney decided to focus on young people at risk, who were part of the Pembury estate. Modelled on the Harlem Children's Zone in New York, the initiative focused on three specific strands: early years and primary, secondary education and, third, support for parents (9). Through a range of projects, including the relocation of a children's centre to the estate, access to child care, breakfast and after school clubs, career advice and adult learning courses, the project aimed at addressing issues of crime and deprivation. It was a partnership between housing, the children's centre, local schools and the youth services and demonstrated how much could be achieved by integration and cooperation.

Two schemes – one in Newcastle and the other in Surrey – worked with groups at opposite ends of the childhood spectrum. In Newcastle the aim was to boost the uptake of two-year-olds receiving child care. The scheme, based on a door-to-door campaign, managed to achieve an increase in uptake from 76% to 92%, through a partnership between Sure Start Children's Centres and childcare providers (9). In Surrey an integrated scheme between local schools, colleges, employers, voluntary organisations and higher education succeeded in improving the attainment in learning and reducing the number of young people not in education and employment training.

Finally, two further examples of integrating parts of children's services are provided by Salford and Devon. Both concern early years' services where arguments for some degree of integration seem to be more easily made. Salford Early Intervention and Prevention Service came into existence in 2011 and aimed to address problems at the earliest opportunity, before they escalate and in partnership with other organisations. The Salford Children's Services Joint Working Protocol was a three-way partnership between the city council, a forum of voluntary, community and social enterprise organisations and Salford community and voluntary services (10). Its bold aims were, amongst other things, to reduce the number of children living in poverty and to improve the health and well-being of children and families.

In a similar vein, the Devon Early Help initiative again aimed at addressing extra needs and preventing situations from getting more difficult for children and young people. Here, however, rather than a designated team, the Devon model operated on the basis that every agency would work together to support the needs of families. So, early help is offered by all organisations that work with children – whether this is youth workers, social workers, support workers, Children's Centres or GPs (11).

The above examples are little more than a random snapshot at attempts at limited integration. They do, however, serve to illustrate how with joined-up approaches to care, progress can be made and the whole is more than the sum of its parts. Bringing social care agencies together whether this is to support specific groups of children in the care system, the unemployed or vulnerable families, helps to demonstrate the benefits of integrated services. There are, however, two significant challenges facing calls for greater integration of social care; the one is specific to local authorities and the other is generic to all attempts at integration.

In relation to the first of these is the wholesale contracting out of services to private and voluntary sector providers we saw in Chapter 6. This makes integration even more of a challenge when what drives development is largely what is or is not in a contract to deliver a specific service.

It is not surprising, therefore, that the Local Government Association, in looking at integration, would concentrate on what it describes as "alternative delivery models" for children's services (12). These include:

- outsourcing or contracting for the delivery of certain aspects of children's services in a local area such as fostering and adoption services;
- joint management teams, where councils join together;
- setting up separate entities, through which services are delivered, such as an independent Children's Trust.

An example of the latter of these can be found in the Doncaster Children's Services Trust, established in 2014. This set up a company limited by guarantee with a board of directors and a director of social services who remained within children's services and is responsible both for commissioning and monitoring services. By contrast, Kingston upon Thames and Richmond upon Thames established a social enterprise company to deliver all educational support and children's social care services, as well as integrated health services for children with disabilities. It might be argued that the social enterprise companies or trusts have more opportunity to integrate services than local authorities who commission services from a range of private providers. As a consequence of the latter, integration becomes more difficult where new transactions or partnerships may not be seen as part of a contract and have to be negotiated separately. Some of these proposals clearly fall in line with the Conservative government's *Putting Children First*, examined in Chapter 3.

These new and emerging patterns for the way services are being delivered need to be kept firmly in mind when we come to propose a new model, in Chapter 8. We cannot ignore the complexity of the present funding landscape. Similarly, and this relates particularly to any integration going beyond social care, we need to be very aware of the challenges of data sharing across multi-professions. Much more will be said about this in Chapter 8, when we come to look at the proposed model. Suffice to say here that Section 10 of the Children Act 2004 places a duty on key people and bodies to cooperate and this includes the sharing of information. It was proposed that there should be information sharing agreements, exchanged on a case by case basis. But real integration involves going further than this and finding new ways to create a common database, used by all relevant agencies.

Multi-Agency Safeguarding Hubs (MASH)

Before turning attention to examples of integration in health, two significant initiatives deserve consideration. The first of these – MASH services – undoubtedly provide the closest we currently have to integration of services for a specific group of children. The second – the Greater Manchester Combined Authority – has the potential for providing a way forward for integration that might be mirrored elsewhere.

Multi-Agency Safeguarding Hubs (MASH) have now been developed in a number of parts of England and take as their starting point the co-location of staff, from a wide variety of professional backgrounds, to provide an integrated approach to child protection. The composition of MASH staff varies but the core is likely to include social workers, education, health and the police with individual hubs also choosing to include probation, the ambulance service, youth justice or housing. What the MASH provide is a single point of entry for child protection enquiries, which might be via letter, emails or telephone calls. They permit the sharing of information between agencies, allow referrals to be triaged, facilitate early intervention and manage cases through rapidly convened multi-agency case discussions.

Once a referral is received there is usually a search of the various databases, to see what is known of the children and carers and to provide the basis for a meeting of all of the agencies who might have an involvement (13). This then allows a decision to be rapidly made as to which should be the lead agency and what action is necessary. MASH teams operate in areas as varied as Devon and London and in some large urban cities like Birmingham. In an early assessment of MASH schemes in London, commissioned by the London Councils, it was agreed that they shared five underlying principles:

- All safeguarding goes through the hub.
- All co-located staff deliver an integrated service.
- The hub is "fire walled", keeping MASH activity confidential and separate from operational activity.
- They have agreed processes to determine the appropriate agency for action.
- They need to develop processes to identify potential and actual victims.

Early evidence from the London MASH hubs indicated that they have the potential to address some of the issues highlighted in serious case reviews from the past and develop more effective multi-agency working. "There are signs that the professionals working together in MASH teams were developing their own MASH culture as distinct from single agency cultures" (14, p. 4). This is most important. The idea that multi-agency working creates a new and shared culture that is different from the culture of a single organisation is a powerful support for this kind of approach. It is a fundamental argument for the establishment of integrated working where the whole is not only greater than the sum of its parts but fundamentally different from the parts themselves. Furthermore, MASH schemes have the potential for improvement in partnership communication and information sharing. The survey also found that the turnaround of cases was reduced, there was better understanding of roles and evidence that children were receiving services appropriate to their needs, following a referral.

A larger, longitudinal study of 37 local authorities with MASH schemes, conducted by the Home Office in 2014, similarly concluded that they all adhered to three principles of (a) information sharing, (b) joint decision making and (c) coordinated intervention (13). Furthermore, and very much as a result of these principles, MASH schemes were able to make more accurate assessments of risk and need, there were consequently fewer repeat referrals, greater efficiencies and more thorough and driven management of the cases.

The physical location of MASH schemes varied from police stations to social services premises, reflecting local priorities. What remains a challenge, however is good integrated IT systems. Most areas lacked this, and many felt that this just wasn't feasible. Instead, information from several sets of different professional databases had to be consulted, in order to arrive at a composite picture of child and family circumstances. And, of course, some health authorities, for example, have more than one IT system under which they operate.

MASH schemes represent the closest we will come to any current integration of children's services. And they are, of course, specific to child protection. But evidence that this degree of inter-professional problem-solving leads to better decisions, a quicker response for children and the forging of a new shared culture that overrides the views of single professions should be borne in mind when we come to explore a wider integrated child care system in Chapter 8.

Creating a new health and care system in Manchester

In February 2015 the then chancellor, George Osborne, launched a plan for devolving health and social care, which had the potential to bring about a fundamental change to the way services were delivered. It was to be part of the Northern Powerhouse initiative, discussed in Chapter 3, and brought together the 15 NHS providers, 10 local authorities and 37 statutory authorities involved in health and social care in Greater Manchester. It established the Greater Manchester Combined Authority, with a £6 billion budget for health and social care; serving a population of 2.8 million people.

Much of the thinking behind this initiative will now be familiar to readers of this book. Care – so the plan asserted (15) – is not joined up between teams. Millions of pounds are annually spent dealing with illness caused by poverty, loneliness, stress, debt, drinking and other social causes. In Greater Manchester a number of key health outcomes were worse than in some other areas of the UK, with too little overall coordination of remedies. The newly constituted combined authority established some early priorities aimed at, amongst other things, creating a unified public health leadership for Greater Manchester and ensuring that everyone had access to primary care services.

It is important to emphasise that the Manchester plan is wider than children's services and also embraces both adult and elderly care. It envisages an enhancement of primary care services with local GPs driving new models of care and Local Care Organisations (LCOs) to include community, social care, acute mental health services, the full range of third sector providers and other local providers such as schools. The plan was to locate LCOs in the places where most people use and access services in their communities and close to home.

What is proposed is not an incremental change, but a fundamental rethinking of the way services across the whole care system are organised. It is a radical set of proposals, attempting to bridge some of the unnecessary splits between health and social care and giving primary care the lead role in how organisations will work collaboratively. As such, it is seeking to answer the needs of the total population.

The chief executive of NHS England described the Manchester plan as having the potential to be the greatest act of devolution there has ever been in the history of the NHS (16). It also fits in with the wider coming together of health and social care, through the more widely developing Sustainability and Transformation Partnerships (STPs) and Integrated Care Systems (ICSs) that are being delivered in England by Clinical Commissioning Groups, to encourage health and social care to work more closely together.

The Manchester experiment has some way to go before its effectiveness can properly be evaluated. Chapter 3, which readers will recall looked at a range of short-term initiatives, would teach us to be cautious about sustainability. But an initiative that takes as its starting point:

- the need for early intervention;
- the knowledge that many health problems are the results of social and economic causes;
- the requirement to bring together statutory services on a scale not previously seen;
- the siting of services at a local level;
- the importance of community engagement in planning.

All have a resonance with the book's main thesis.

Achieving greater integration within health services

It is not surprising that the calls for greater integration of social services are also mirrored in health. Wolfe et al. make reference to the unsatisfactory healthcare experiences of families, such as multiple appointments for children both in different locations and on different days and inadequate coordination and communication between professionals, also noted in Chapter 1. Their solution, specifically in relation to the health service is:

> Comprehensive integrated teams in primary care settings should provide the majority of children's healthcare . . . The teams should comprise jointly trained general practitioners and paediatricians working with children's nurses, health visitors allied health professionals and mental health professionals.
>
> *(17, p. 903)*

Such teams could provide high quality urgent care for minor illness, preventing the need for unnecessary referrals or hospital admissions.

Roy Lilley went further, suggesting that primary care delivered by GPs will need to change:

> The practice unit will have to go the way of the corner shop. Today's chaotic care where patients are bounced between primary and secondary care, social services and the support agencies has to end. The interfaces are wasteful and the results haphazard.
>
> *(18, p. 2)*

Of course, he is writing of adult services as well. However, an NCB report echoed the same theme, specifically in relation to children's health and argued that while a lot of the more specialist expertise in many areas of child health is based on secondary care providers, it really needs to be in general practice. This would reduce hospital admissions and allow more children to be treated in the community (19). GPs should be supported by specialists and those trained in child health. The idea of general practice as a focal point for integrated children's services is – like the idea of social care hubs – one to which we will return in Chapter 8.

Similarly, in relation to integrated health services, the BMA concluded, in 2013, that:

> Children's services and the structures that enable them, should be coordinated in the interests of children and families. This will require financial and organisational coordination, supportive local and national policy and adequate resources, invested for sufficient time to enable improvement.
>
> *(20, p. 33)*

This latter point about allowing sufficient time to embed change and permit it to be properly evaluated takes us straight back to arguments about short-term projects, rapidly replaced by other equally short-term initiatives, which we examined in Chapter 3.

Lastly, in terms of calls for integrated health services for children, Sir Ian Kennedy in his report on children's health services, reached similar conclusions, pointing to the lack of coordination between services, the "complex array and interplay of organisations, units and teams and the way in which the NHS failed to join up with other services" (21, p. 13).

Kennedy particularly highlighted the problem for young people in transition between children and adult services. For his Inquiry it was not simply a failure between health and social care: education was often excluded from "joined up thinking". In the criminal justice system strong links between the police and NHS staff were often lacking and local organisations failed to work together:

> Whatever the precise structural mechanism, there should be an organisation for every area (perhaps coterminous with that of the Local Authority) dedicated

> wholly to meeting the needs of children and young people, and which exists to bring local public services together in order to do this.
>
> *(21, p. 9)*

In an attempt to overcome some of the silo thinking that has sometimes characterised health, as it has social services, there have been a number of new and emerging models of care. Again, these examples are illustrative and certainly not exhaustive.

The Nuffield Trust has recorded a scheme in North West London, where between two to six GP practices work with paediatric consultants to provide care to practice populations of approximately 4,000 children. GPs in these hub practices discuss cases, hold multi-disciplinary meetings and provide enhanced support within their host communities (22).

A children and young people's health partnership, based on the Evelina Children's Hospital, focuses on the everyday health (and includes social care) for a population of 120,000 children and young people in the London boroughs of Southwark and Lambeth. It represents a coalition of the local Clinical Commissioning Groups, local authorities, acute providers, the voluntary sector and family and patient representatives. The scheme has focused on four major components:

- "a whole system approach" for children and young people experiencing long-term conditions;
- the improvement of everyday healthcare, including joint clinics and training between GPs and paediatrics;
- improving access to services, including the active engagement of users in any planning; and
- cross-system training, to increase shared understanding of differing roles.

(22)

Although originating in health, in an area serving very diverse inner London communities, it can be seen how this model seeks to draw in other professional disciplines.

A third example of efforts to improve health integration, and again recorded by the Nuffield Trust, is the Liverpool Family Health and Wellbeing model. This sought to establish a multi-agency culture of shared care and seamless delivery across child and family services. Once more, the aim of this model was clinicians from primary and secondary care working both together and closer to local authority colleagues. All of this joint working aimed to achieve better paediatric services in the community, better links with other professionals and a more systematic approach to early intervention.

A final, and slightly unusual, example of integration concerns a link between special educational needs co-coordinators (SENCOs) and GPs in Barnstaple. Four medical centres had linked with local schools and SENCOs to provide a more holistic service for children and young people with special needs. This included an educational psychology session focussing on attachment and anxiety in young people, medical centres writing to schools outlining the process and support for facilitating joint working and one of the medical practices nominating a partner to lead on communication with schools. As the project concluded "there is clear evidence that joint working is enabling more targeted care to be provided and all professionals have a better understanding of the child's and parent's needs" (23, p.1).

International patterns of child care

A glance at what happens to the integration of services for children and young people in other countries not only helps provide comparisons with UK practice but also a fresh perspective. However, it needs acknowledging that this is inevitably a very brief, paper-based exercise, calling on the research of organisations like Eurochild. The subject deserves a whole book to itself.

C4EO provides a useful starting point, having looked not only at the delivery of children's service in other parts of the world, but the policy context within which they operate (24). This compares child care in Nordic countries (Denmark, Finland, Iceland, Norway and Sweden and also the Netherlands) with English-speaking and American practice. The paper begins by examining some of the international data we considered in Chapter 4. Generally, the Nordic countries ranked highly on international indicators of material well-being, housing and the environment, educational well-being and health and safety for children. They tend to have comprehensive welfare systems with greater levels of income redistribution than some other European countries.

If we turn specifically to the issue of child protection, C4EO argues that English-speaking countries assume:

> an individualistic or moralistic approach to child abuse problems, the first interventions are legalistic in nature, the relationship between the state and family is marked by conflict and thus placements are made primarily against the will of the family.
>
> *(24, n.p.)*

In comparison, Nordic countries adopt what is described as a family service orientation and a "social or psychological" approach to child abuse. The first interventions are focused on the needs of the family and the expectations are that interventions will take place at the least formal level: in other words, within local communities and with state help available if necessary. Compare this with the United States and what C4EO describes as a "reactive" approach to child welfare – with a limited role for the state and intervention only when the need is explicit. It is noticeable that in the States there are separate federal departments of education, health and human services.

What we sometimes find in several European countries is, first, the concept of "pedagogy" (which is in some ways a statement about integration) and, second, the integration of services at a national level. Still relatively unfamiliar in the UK, pedagogy represents some coming together of education and social care. Basic training in pedagogy combines education with what is sometimes described as "upbringing". Pedagogues are trained in child development and work therapeutically with children and families in a wide range of settings. It is firmly based in education and uses educational methods to treat social ills. Although it has evolved differently in different European countries, it includes both the social and intellectual environment and has a fundamental focus on the care and well-being of the child, teaching social skills and cultural norms. It will now be seen that this bringing together of education with some aspects of social care represents a kind of integration within one professional group.

The second characteristic, in some countries, is a much closer integration of government departments, responsible for children. In the Netherlands, for example, the Ministry of Youth and Families was created in 2007, as an "umbrella" ministry within which four ministries operate – the Ministry of Health, Welfare and Sport, the Ministry of Justice, the Ministry of Education, Culture and Science and the Ministry of Social Affairs and Employment. Confronted with the situation of an increase in children with behavioural problems, of young people who attended neither school nor work and a surge in anti-social behaviour, it was felt there was a need for concerted collaborative close working relationships between ministries, the municipal and provincial authorities, youth care institutes, schools and other stakeholders as the only way to tackle such problems. One example of this was the Brede School Initiative in the Netherlands, where schools work with a range of agencies including the police, health and welfare services, sports and cultural institutions to enhance pupils' opportunities for development. And to be successful, integration needs to start at the top amongst government ministries.

Two further papers also help to illustrate how integrated practice differs both in other parts of Europe and other parts of the world. Hosking et al. examine the premise that early intervention increases the chance of the best outcomes and provides integrated examples of this from around the world (25). These examples are illustrative:

1. Stop ACES, Oneida County, New York USA looked at the effects of adverse childhood experiences on the long-term "well-being" of young people. Drawing on the health, education and mental health departments in the county, the project developed strategies and interventions to promote positive parenting – in order to counteract earlier experiences.
2. A second American project, CASASTART (Striving Together to Achieve Rewarding Tomorrows), was designed to keep high-risk 8–13-year-olds free of drugs and involvement in crime. It represented a partnership between youth and youth justice, schools and after school programmes.
3. The Eve Family Initiative programme in South Brisbane in Australia was established as a preventive programme to forestall the development of mental health problems in children. It targeted parents of four- to seven-year-old children making the transition to primary school and included a range of

services from GPs to other health workers and the education sector. The emphasis on all three of these schemes is both early intervention and the need for a multi-disciplinary approach to complex child and family challenges.

In a similar vein, Eurochild published what was described as a "Compendium of Inspiring Practices", looking at examples of early intervention and prevention for children across Europe. They established five criteria that underpinned all of the considered family and support services:

- frame family policy within a child's rights approach;
- recognise and respect diversity in family patterns;
- respect children's rights to be heard;
- take a strength-based approach and remain non-judgemental;
- provide universally accessible support, which reaches those in greatest need.

and added that all examples demonstrate "inter-service collaboration" as a way of engaging with families, building their resilience and empowering them. In many of the examples quoted, integration goes further than collaboration and constructively involves services working together. Examples from Eurochild include:

- An imaginative scheme in Flanders and Brussels, Belgium, led to the establishment of Parenting Shops, creating the opportunity for organisations to come together to deliver services to parents, as a co-ordinated and integrated package, accessible to every parent. Not only do the shops offer information to parents, but also counselling and education and training activities. Other parenting support can be offered in other locations, such as schools or community centres. Everyone involved in the parenting of children aged 0–18 are welcome to use the shops, which call upon a range of agencies to offer help and advice.
- What is particularly noticeable from the Eurochild "compendium" is the wide range of locations within which preventive services are located. In the federal state of North Rhine–Westphalia, Germany, a scheme to turn the 9,000 child-care centres into family centres is not dissimilar to the UK's Sure Start initiative. The aim was to achieve easy accessibility to families for support, with staffing provided by counselling agencies and other professions such a healthcare. While the children's centres were the central hub, "hard to reach families" were visited at home and other locations imaginatively included local libraries, retirement homes for the elderly and sports clubs – providing activities for children.
- In the Good Parent–Good Start project in Warsaw, Poland, the location was local health centres, as all parents have to register their newborn children there. This provided both a universal and targeted service aimed at preventing the abuse of children under six. The project operated at four levels,

starting with information on parenting to intervention in cases of child abuse. To begin with, the scheme aimed at families either expecting a child or with one from 0–3 and then extended to include four- to six-year-olds.

- Similar to the German scheme, a project in Italy, aimed at "mother–child" family units at high risk of social or psychological distress during the first year of their child's life, based activities in the family home. It was deliberately focused on carers of "low educational level", single parents, those experiencing drug problems or those of immigrant status. It provided programmes to support the mother–child relationship and adopted a multi-disciplinary approach, drawing in obstetric and neonatology staff from wards of the city's hospitals.
- Lastly, and very different was a Spanish project – Bultzatzen – Promoting Success, based in the Basque country. It deliberately targeted young people aged 12–16 at risk of academic failure and social exclusion. Help has involved the family, community, schools, the town council, university and other institutions. Based on the already quoted belief that it takes a whole village to raise a child, it tried to engage not just teachers but the whole community, covering out-of-school hours and involving a network of agencies including social services and "socio-educational teams". The location was wherever space existed with other community activities, women's group meeting places and adult schools or kindergarten.

(26)

A number of common strands will be evident from the above examples. First, an overriding emphasis on prevention in the hope that this would help deal with social and emotional pressures before they escalate. Second, the emphasis on using a wide variety of locations, from homes to community centres, in order to reach out to families. Third, and this will come as no surprise, the need for a whole range of professionals to be involved. As a final example, a scheme in Finland illustrates how far-reaching inter-disciplinary working can be.

On Finland's border with Russia the local maternity clinic had been merged with family services. As a result of a routine pregnancy check-up, staff were alerted to the plight of a pregnant woman with four children from a husband who had now abandoned her. She had no car, had difficulty walking and was struggling to cope. The newly combined service provided healthcare, shopping, cleaning, day care, navigated the bureaucracy of income support and provided help to strengthen her parenting skills. For this and similar situations the team had seen themselves moving from child protection to preventive work. As one worker remarked: "When you have a multi-disciplinary group you have to talk to other professionals, even if you are not sure what you are saying is right" (27, p. 40).

And, as we saw earlier, there is then the possibility that a corporate culture is created from an amalgamation of the various professions involved, focused not on one approach but the holistic needs of children.

The meaning of integration

We began this chapter by describing integration as an aerosol term. Indeed, this chapter pleads guilty to discussing integration while also not having defined it clearly. If we are to propose a new model for the way that children's services could be delivered across health, social care, housing, the voluntary sector and recreation etc., then we need to be more disciplined in outlining what integration *really* is and how its effectiveness might be evaluated. These criteria can then be taken into Chapter 8, to evaluate the robustness of the proposed new model.

Some of the most helpful work on a disciplined meaning of integration, particularly in relation to paediatric services, has been done by the British Association of Community Child Health (BACCH) (28). While the outcome of any integration should always be "seamless, smooth and easy to navigate" (p. 3) services, BACCH argues that this can take many different forms. First, is what they describe as organisational integration or merger, where two or more organisations become one. Second, at a lesser level, integration can involve the coming together of the finance or other functions, such as human resources or the services themselves. So, in relation to the latter, we have the various efforts to combine clinical services. Third, and in recent years we have seen several attempts to achieve this, the combining of IT or information systems; sometimes with the hope that if the databases are joined the rest of the organisations will reluctantly or willingly follow. Lastly, is what BACCH defines as workforce integration, where employers combine under one of the existing organisations or even form a new one.

Equally important are the *principles* hat lie behind successful integration. Here lie some of the metrics against which success or failure can be judged. To be successful, BACCH argues, integration needs to achieve the following:

- It should be "patient" or client focused, concentrating on the needs of the individual.
- It should mean integration across the whole pathways – so that there should be improved access to a range of services, in a timely manner.
- The geographical/population coverage should be such that all individuals can benefit equally.
- It should lead to quality improvement, which should be part of a continuous process.
- The information systems and data should enhance communication across the whole pathway.
- There should be shared values and leadership, leading to a cohesive and joined-up culture.
- Stakeholders/patients /clients should be actively engaged in both planning and improving the services.
- There should be strong accountability through a clear governance structure.
- Funding and financial management must promote inter-professional teamwork.
- It should have political support to succeed.
- There should be a workforce which shares the same values.

As BACCH concludes, integration is challenging if it is to achieve improvement in prevention, cure and rehabilitation. The distinction between varying types of integration and their key principles should serve us well as we turn to what an integrated child care system might truly mean. For as the Social Care Institute for Excellence concluded: "Working in collaboration is essential if individuals are to be offered the range of support they require in a timely manner. Multi-agency working is about providing a seamless response to individuals with multiple and complex needs" (29, p. 1).

Notes

1 *Multiple needs. Time for political leadership*. Clinks and Mind, 2017.
2 *It takes a village and other lessons children teach us*. Clinton, H.R., 1996, Simon and Schuster, New York.
3 *The Team around the Child (TAC) and the lead professional. A guide for practitioners*. The Children's Workforce Development Council, 2009. Supported by the Department for Children, Schools and Families, Children's Workforce Development Council, Leeds.
4 *Rewiring public services, our ambition for children and young people*. 2013, Local Government Association.
5 *These are our children*. A review by Dame Christine Lenehan into the care of children with learning disabilities. Department of Health and Social Care, 2017.
6 *Tired all the time. The impact of sleep difficulties on families with disabled children*. The Family Fund, 2013, York.
7 *Making Britain great for children and families*. 4Children, 2014, London.
8 *Evaluation of the no wrong door innovation programme*. Lushey, C., Hyde-Dryden, G., Holmes, L. and Blackmore, T., 2017, Department of Education.
9 See *State of the nation 2017: social mobility in Great Britain*. Social Mobility Commission, 2017.
10 *Salford children's services joint working protocol with voluntary and community organisations and social enterprises*. Salford City Council, undated.
11 *Early help in Devon*. Devon Children and Families Partnership, 2017.
12 *Scrutinising alternative delivery models for children's services*. Centre for Public Scrutiny and Local Government Association, November 2017.
13 *Multi-agency working and information sharing project*. Final Report. Home Office, July 2014.
14 *Assessing the early impact of Multi-Agency Safeguarding Hubs (MASH) in London*. Crockett, R., Gilchrist, G., Davies, J., Henshall, A., Hoggart, L., Chandler, V., Simms, V. and Webb, J., 2013, Commissioned by the London Councils.
15 *Taking charge of our health and social care in Greater Manchester*. Greater Manchester Combined Authority 2015.
16 Quoted in *The Guardian*, Tuesday 24 March 2015.
17 How can we improve child health services? Wolfe, I. et al., *British Medical Journal*, 2011, 23 April, vol 342, 901–904.
18 *The value we can extract*. Lilley, R., 2013, NHS Managers.
19 *Opening the door to better healthcare: ensuring general practice is working for children and young people*. Clements, K., 2013, National Children's Bureau, London.
20 *Growing up in the UK. Ensuring a healthy future for our children*. BMA Board of Science, 2013, London.
21 *Getting it right for children and young people: overcoming cultural barriers in the NHS so as to meet their needs*. Kennedy, Professor Sir Ian, 2016, Department of Health and Social Care.
22 This example, together with that of the Evelina Children's Hospital and the Liverpool Family Health and Wellbeing model are to be found in *The future of child health services: new models of care*. Kossarova, L., Devakukmar, D. and Edwards, N., 2016, Nuffield Trust.

23 *Devon SEND good practice example GP/SENCO's collaborative working*. Undated. Devon County Council.
24 *Delivering children's services in the UK and other parts of the world – a short policy context.* C4EO, August 2011, London.
25 *International experience of early intervention for children, young people and their families.* Hosking, G. and Walsh, I., 2010, The Wave Trust, Croydon.
26 *Early intervention and prevention in family and parenting support.* Compendium of Inspiring Practices, Eurochild, October 2012.
27 Finland is pioneering joined-up services and reaping the rewards. Crouch, D., 2015, *The Guardian*, Wednesday 9 September.
28 *The meaning of "integrated care" for children and families in the UK.* British Association of Community Child Health. Position Statement, 2012, London.
29 *Multi agency working. Outcome statement 10*, SCIE NQSW resource, 2010, SCIE Publications, London.

8

BUILDING A WORLD CLASS CHILDREN'S SERVICE

Some key principles

Sir Anthony Panizzi was forthright in arguing for a new London-based national library. "The expense will no doubt be great", he asserted "but so is the nation which is to bear it". The chutzpah worked, and the "great" nation went ahead and built the British Library. The same "great" UK has a deserved reputation for providing services for children. We have seen charities give way to the welfare state. David Lloyd George's promise that after the First World War there would be "a fit country for heroes to live in" and the Beveridge proposals, were to provide jobs and houses for those returning from the war: leading, first, to the modern NHS and a gradual diversification of providers of services for children. This diversification is the case whether you look at health, social care, education, and housing or leisure services. But are we now ready to "bear" the expense of a world class children's service?

The Seebohm report imagined a "family centred", rather than a "symptom-centred" service, with one door through which all social problems would haltingly march. But Seebohm saw the solution more narrowly than is proposed here and largely in terms of local authority services. This did not include integration with health or housing or even with the voluntary sector. We have now reached a point where integration for children's services needs to take place on a scale not previously seen. It will mean a programme that could take 20 years to implement, will require wide political support and cannot be seen as yet another fleeting initiative, to be replaced by the next short-term solution.

To achieve this means creating fundamentally new relationships between providers of children's social care, health, education, housing, youth services, employment, the voluntary sector, police, leisure and the private sector. It requires a sea-change in thinking, unprecedented since the 1940s Beveridge reforms.

But the arguments are overwhelming. Only by looking holistically at a child's needs and engaging all of the agencies can these needs be met. There is little point in repeatedly patching up a child with asthma and a serious chest condition in an A&E department, if he is going to be returned to a damp, cold and polluted house. There is little point in trying to educate an academically struggling young carer if her mind and worried emotions are permanently focused at school on the disabled mother back at home for whom she has principal responsibility. And there is little point in putting the family of a disabled child through the merry-go-round of numerous medical specialists, none of whom have contact or liaise with each other.

Integration – on the scale outlined below – should have a series of principles that supplement those defined by BACCH in Chapter 7:

- It should pre-eminently be child focused, turning "wraparound care" from a slogan to a reality.
- It should reflect the *zeitgeist* of "localism", embraced by the major political parties and fit in with the demographics of a specific neighbourhood.
- It needs to reflect the complexity of the present funding environment – with state, voluntary and private sector providers.
- It should encompass health, social care, education, leisure, youth services, police, housing, the voluntary and private sectors and the benefit agencies.
- It should have a genuinely preventive agenda, aiming to intervene early to stop problems developing.
- It should function according to the pyramid of need, outlined in Chapter 1, where those in greatest need receive the most support.
- It should not involve another major re-organisation of any single specialism.

Three of the principles listed above – localism, the complexity of the present funding environment and the avoidance of further major re-organisation – require more elucidation.

Localism

Any proposed children and young person's service needs to recognise the growing appetite for what is increasingly described as "localism". So, the demands of, say, an isolated rural community where transport may be a permanent problem, employment limited and towns dispersed, will not be the same as what is needed in inner city areas. Inner city Birmingham will be very different from rural Devon or Suffolk or seaside towns like Weston-super-Mare. The coming together of new patterns of services needs to begin with an acknowledgement of this. At the same time it makes sense to keep any new structure aligned with the present system of local government.

Second, there needs to be a recognition that there is now a wealth of providers of children's services, each contributing to the mix of care as outlined in Chapter 6. So, for example, support to young people leaving care may be contracted out to a large voluntary organisation such as Barnardo's or Action for Children or services might be commissioned to one of the major private sector providers. A model that does not recognise this will fall at the first hurdle.

At the same time, the new structure would allow a much tighter and more coherent system for integrating voluntary and private sector providers into a coherent, holistic service. Nothing will stop voluntary organisations running services that consist entirely of voluntary funding, i.e. the money they raise themselves. Although, even here, it is to be hoped that planned new services will be agreed at a local level, by the CST board (see below), to fit in with the district's overall strategic vision. In the case of directly contracted services there should be a greater sense of ownership by all the combined integrated services and more awareness as to how they contribute to the overall needs of the children's population.

Third, in terms of re-organisation, the proposed Children's Services Teams (CSTs) have, as their starting point, the allocation of staff from health, social care, education, leisure, housing etc. into a new multi-disciplinary team. But it is not about forging a single organisation or department in which all of the professional groups take on new identities. Instead, health visitors, for example, would continue to be employed by the NHS and still gain their professional training or validation from their own professional bodies. It is *not* about creating new, rigid roles but a model that permits separate professional groups to come together and allocate staff in a way that directly reflects local needs. It is closer to a secondment, in which multi-disciplinary staff work within the umbrella of the CST. Very much in line with some of the Multi-Agency Safeguarding Hubs, described in Chapter 7.

If we return to the series of principles, outlined by BACCH in Chapter 7, it will be seen that what is proposed is not a new system in which a whole range of organisations become one. Instead, it is closer to what BACCH outlined as "workforce integration" in which staff mix within a common team, while remaining part of, say, the NHS, social care or the voluntary organisation which employs them.

Lastly, the integration of children's services is not about a single, prescribed model; it would very much be a reflection of local circumstances and requirements as to how the new organisation was configured. More of this will be discussed below. What the rest of this chapter will do is, firstly, to outline the model in more detail and, secondly, describe how it would work.

Children's services teams (CSTs)

Each locality will have a multidisciplinary CST. It will serve differing size populations, very much dependent on whether it is based in a rural or urban area. It will be up to the local CST management board (see below) to determine population size for a CST. This will be based on existing local government and health teams, district, town or city structures and a workable, good fit with existing organisations. Each locality will have a central CST administrative and operational base, where professionals working across the whole spectrum of prevention, support and help for children will come together. This will include representatives of primary care, health visitors, district nurses, community paediatricians, children's social workers, school representatives, voluntary and private sector providers of services, housing and housing association workers, school nurses, occupational and speech therapists, CAMHS staff, those involved in income support, the police and youth justice services and those who run local leisure services for children.

Professionals attached to the CSTs will form two distinct groups – those who are full-time CST team members, such as community paediatricians, children's social workers, educational support liaison workers and health visitors. Second, those for whom engagement will be on a part-time basis, such as housing, leisure or income support workers. The latter group may also have responsibilities in relation to adult care and will therefore be brought in when additional support services or professional expertise for children and their families is required.

Bringing teams of disparate professionals together is not without considerable challenge. For example, a locality CST team will realistically not be able to include representatives from each school or GP practice as members of the CST team. There will need to be some system of delegation in which individuals represent their wider constituency. They will then take on the responsibility to both refer children to the central team and take back any recommendations and actions to ensure they are implemented. At the same time it is proposed that when there are serious child protection concerns for a child and family, then the GP and school, for example, will be fully represented. (This will involve a much greater use of Skype/video conferencing technology etc. See below.) However, it is important to note that the CST are operational and not strategic units (very much like the MASH teams); so discussion and decision will be at the level of what intervention might be best for a specific child. Strategy within a CST locality will be determined by the board.

The engagement of GPs is particularly challenging. On average, members of the public see their GP six times a year; double the number of visits from a decade ago (1). Surprisingly, as Chapter 4 highlighted, many GPs receive little training in child health and their working lives make it difficult, for example, under present arrangements to engage in child protection case conferences. Also, it is highly likely that the new CSTs will cut across several GP practices. But two factors in the new arrangements should help to engage GPs more closely in the new structure.

First, the bringing together of a range of professionals within the same virtual team will mean that the kind of holistic approach to a child and the many dimensions to his or her life – which conscientious GPs often know – should now be available to the whole team. Second, either collectively or individually, GP practices will nominate a representative who will be part of the overall CST team; feeding into discussions and concerns about specific children and their carers and contributing to any case plan. The greater contribution of GPs is absolutely vital to the success of CSTs.

The location of CSTs

The location of CSTs is challenging, with a number of potential solutions. The model proposes that they will become focal points within their local communities.

In this context one of the strengths of the Extended Schools initiative, explored in Chapter 3 was the reality that schools are non-stigmatising environments –since most of the young population attend schools. Large schools with the necessary space could provide an attractive location for CSTs and would have an immediate link with many of the children who require additional support and are educated in the state sector.

Equally free from stigma are GP health centres, which increasingly combine a range of functions such as clinics, support groups, crèches and other services. Where such centres are coming together to combine practices there could be some capacity for the location of a local CST; and, of course, other nursing staff such as midwives and nurses may operate from GP practices as well.

Alongside health centres as possible CST locations are the "one-stop shops" developed by some local authorities where libraries, community policing, health clinics and housing, for example, operate from the same public facing building. However, more realistically, the solution may lie in newly built or adapted buildings, capable of accommodating the multidisciplinary CST teams. Space will be needed for baby clinics, interview and consultancy rooms for social workers and paediatricians to examine children, interview suites for the investigation of child abuse and space for advice sessions for housing or income support to take place. Ensuring that CST centres are also where the new babies and their carers were registered, would ensure that there was an initial contact with all newborns. The ideal would be purpose-built centres, designed with children in mind, with reception desks at child height, toys much in evidence and a welcoming, friendly environment, conducive to warm interactions between children, carers and professionals. It is so often the case that public facing – public sector – buildings for children are inferior to the kind of design and décor we automatically expect of the private sector. CSTs present a real opportunity to ensure that we build something different – with the same high standards we expect from private sector services. The vision is of a national network of CST child-centred buildings, welcoming to families and attractive places in which to work. To treat people with respect and dignity is to heighten the possibility of this being reciprocated.

It is further proposed that the CST would operate a hub and spokes model. As well as the central location of the team in a single place would be spokes, or sub-offices, where for, example, babies could be weighed or young people interviewed. Essential to the success of the CST will be both their accessibility to the local population and the close working relationship between the hub and these spokes. In rural areas, where populations are dispersed, the spokes will be vital to ensure people can engage with CST members, connected to good IT and communication facilities.

Four further elements are essential to the introduction of the CST model; pooled budgets, a common referral and assessment process, the allocation of a Named Person who principally works with the child and lastly, the development of a technology that would securely allow both the exchange of information and better diagnostic and treatment tools.

CST budgets and the assessment process

Pooling budgets is essential to the CST model. The idea is not new and was proposed, in relation to the development of Sure Start centres. The All Party Parliamentary Sure Start Group called upon local authorities, Health and Wellbeing Boards and their local partners to make greater use of pooled budgets to allow for more innovative commissioning of perinatal and children's centre services. Pooled budgets, they argued, would allow a more holistic and preventive approach to working with families, particularly when finances were tight (2). The alternative – a continuation of separate funding streams – just creates a silo mentality in which departments hang on to budgets, to conserve resources. Pooled budgets for the CSTs will allow for the commissioning of additional services that the localities feel to be necessary. These pooled budgets will then allow the CST board to buy into additional voluntary or private sector services, needed to respond to specific needs, e.g. a leaving care service or speech and language therapy

The essential starting point for any integrated children's service has to be a *comprehensive* and *shared* referral and assessment process. This, unfortunately, has numerous unsatisfactory precedents. Every Child Matters (3) advocated a standardised approach to conducting assessments of children's needs and deciding how these should be met. It was known as the Common Assessment Framework (CAF) and had three elements consisting of the development of the child or young person, parents and carers and, lastly, the family and environment. The aim was to reduce the number of separate assessments undertaken on children and the kind of duplication described in Chapter 1 in relation, for example, to the Clarence family.

It will come as no surprise to readers to learn that, in 2015, the CAF was superseded by the Early Help Assessment (EHA). One criticism of the CAF was its length and a process that practitioners felt was bureaucratic rather than constructive. This provides a salutary lesson for the assessment process proposed here for CSTs. It is proposed that the referral assessment would consist of two parts – a mix of generic information in Part 1 and specialist in Part 2.

Part 1 will contain generic data, collected for all children. The prize – well worth fighting for – will be a relatively simple assessment form, utilised by a wide range of differing agencies and utilizing generic data available to all. (Clearly, data protection protocols for ensuring that consent had been provided for sharing this common information would need to be properly obtained.) Generic data will include referral details, the source of the referral, the Named Person (see below), child protection issues, domains to be addressed, private or voluntary sector support and the likely duration of any involvement. Examples of Part 1 can be found in the Appendix case studies. It will be noted that the initial referral form also requires information both about the child's level of need and the domains of his or her life to be addressed.

Readers will recall the fourfold pyramid of need, outlined in Chapter 1. This helps to fix the tier of intervention, in terms of intensive help, medium support or signposting to low level services:

- Tier 1 Universal services.
- Tier 2 Additional support needed, e.g. parenting programmes, speech and language help.
- Tier 3 Specialist services, e.g. disability, mental health, school exclusion, offending behaviour, homelessness.
- Tier 4 High dependency, e.g. child with a life-threatening condition.

Doing this as a multi-disciplinary team will be tricky but essential. Each professional group will have its own pyramid of need, which will differ. In social care, for example, prioritisation is linked to what are known as "thresholds", each triggering a different level of services. Here, the thresholds are partly a reflection of local need and resources, ensuring children are free from harm and that childcare law is being followed. The importance of the CST arriving, collectively, at a shared tier of the pyramid is a reminder of one of the conclusions from the MASH teams' research. Here, it was found that inter-agency working eventually overrode the priorities of a single profession.

This becomes evident if we return to the example of the young boy who arrives at his local A&E department with severe asthma and respiratory problems. His breathing difficulties makes him a high priority for the consultant who sees from previous records that there have been several similar admissions to the unit for the same reason. The consultant may have little time to get behind this pattern of admissions, but it could be the case that the boy lives in damp, cold temporary accommodation in a low-income family with a history of unemployment and dependence on state benefits. As a result of the asthma he sometimes misses school and is beginning to fall behind the educational attainment of his peers. But where does the family sit in the housing department's categorisation of need? And how does his poor educational performance compare with that of other children? A multidisciplinary approach, which begins with a shared referral and assessment process, provides a real opportunity to deal with the family's needs holistically and arrive at a consensus about the level of intervention necessary. However, and to repeat, we must not underestimate the challenge of reaching some shared understanding of where top priorities for need, and therefore intervention, may lie.

Lastly, in terms of the shared assessment, is the requirement to provide a simple but comprehensive "taxonomy of need". The Dartington Research Unit define "need" simply as an issue that, if not addressed, will negatively affect a child's normal development. Researchers developed a fivefold classification that encapsulates the major areas of need that require addressing to reach an holistic assessment:

(a) Living situation
(b) Family and social relations
(c) Social and anti-social behaviour
(d) Physical and psychological health
(e) Education and employment.

(4)

Each of these "touch points" need addressing if a child is to be assessed holistically, even if only one or two of them become focused areas of work. (The case studies illustrate just how this would work).

Part 2 of the referral procedure would consist of specific and detailed case information, unique to one of the CST professions. An example of this might be medical information collected by a community paediatrician related to a condition like spina bifida. It would not need to be seen by all CST members but would be essential for an holistic view of the child's overall needs and for specific medical treatment prescribed by the doctor.

A common database and triage system

Equally important as the need for a shared assessment is the requirement to build an electronic recording system, accessed by all CST team members. It needs to be acknowledged that the technology will have to be harnessed on a scale not previously attained. Unfortunately, the track record, either for the NHS or for electronic case recording in social services, is not good. Usually, it has been defeated by a combination of complexity and cost. NHS patient recording systems, for example, have promised much and delivered far less and a previous scheme to introduce standardised electronic recording systems for case records in social services was eventually abandoned. The All Parliamentary Sure Start Group, as well as calling for pooled budgets, could see the need for shared client data and in its recommendations called for "the systematic sharing of live birth data and other appropriate information between health and children's centres" (2, p. 7).

New technology has only slowly been used by the caring professions; partly because the financial investment was seen as difficult to justify when placed against providing direct services for patients or clients. What is now being proposed is more far ranging and absolutely core to the whole existence of CST teams. It means the introduction of a system that would serve the requirements of a number of agencies. It will need to contain generic and specific information that permits a decision to be made as to where a child's needs can best be met. It should have prompts that signpost towards the consideration of other options or pathways that may not have been initially considered. It will also permit the storing of specific data relevant to a particular discipline – what has been described above as Part 2 of the assessment.

It is important to stress the importance of ensuring that the database can access local information. For example, a family where a newborn child has been newly diagnosed with a physical or mental disability may want to find out about local support groups. The work of the Family Fund, which makes annual grants to low-income families with disabled children, points to the way in which the knowledge of other helpful local resources, is often lacking from health and social care agencies. In order to provide a first-class digital system, it will need to be both current and constantly updated. Some of the aps for doctors, outlining pathways of treatment provide a useful comparison for up to date practical assistance.

It needs acknowledging that establishing a shared database for CSTs will present one of the largest challenges for the success of an integrated children's care system. The MASH projects have had limited success in joining databases and it will take a transformational effort if it is to succeed. There is also the need for additional technology to ensure that hubs and spokes can communicate freely, video and skype facilities (for case conferences etc.) should be readily available and CST team members will need up-to-date handheld devices in order to access and add to case note files. To misquote Sir Anthony Panizzi, the expense will no doubt be great but an effective, secure IT system, accessed by a range of agencies, will go a fair distance towards good interagency working.

Referrals and the Named Person

Having established the basis of a common assessment process, which feeds into the shared integrated database, it then becomes necessary to devise a system for the CSTs to receive referrals. It is assumed that these will come into the CST through direct referral (which will mean the CST has to maintain a duty system) or notification from other agencies via email or telephone, letter or personal contact. Each referral should be triaged by three different professions, within the CST, in order to decide what the Common Assessment Framework refers to as the "lead professional role" and we are calling the "Named Person", as established in Scottish legislation. The Named Person not only assumes overall responsibility for ensuring the needs of a child are met, but also becomes the principal point of contact. Such a post was established in Scotland, in 2017 following the introduction of the 2014 Children and Young People (Scotland) Act, with a Named Person (NP) for every child. For many children on tier 1 and in receipt of universal services this would simply be the school head or class teacher, but for children with health, education or social care needs, such a role takes on a much greater importance. The NP is not a guardian but becomes the main person who would not only respond to a child's needs, from the perspective of his or her discipline, but coordinate other services that may be needed and permit a seamless range of support. If we listen to the strong messages that, for example, came from the Clarence family in Chapter 1, there is an established case for a Named Person or professional who would fulfil this service and coordinating role and who is directly responsible to the management of the CST itself.

Another reason for an effective digitally enabled workforce, with an NP and common, shared data is that it will end the lack of coordination evidenced in most child protection investigation reports, since Maria Colwell in 1974. Now with the proposed CST teams, it would be possible to achieve a greater degree of coordination between agencies. In a very real sense child protection would become "everyone's business" with, for example, education, health, social care and the police co-located in the CST hub and more able to become engaged, coordinated by the NP.

Managing the CST

It will also be necessary for each CST to have a nominated head and it is proposed that this would be a statutory function, determined locally. So s/he may come from a range of disciplines (for example, health, social care or education represented within the central team), and this may well differ from area to area. The head's role would not only be to ensure that the team functioned effectively but also to manage the day-to-day administration and produce an annual plan of work. The head would also carry the major responsibility for commissioning additional or main stream services from voluntary and private sector providers.

The head of the CST would be responsible to a Local Management Board, made up of health, social care, education and other statutory providers, together with stakeholders and community representatives. It would be important that public health representatives were fully engaged on the management board, in order to advise on national and local demographic, social and health trends. It would not, however, include private or voluntary sector providers who were commissioned to run services from the CST. There would be an expectation that both the Clinical Commissioning Group and the local authorities would be members of the board. Not only would the board hold the CST head to account but produce a published annual report. This, again, would be a statutory document that reflected a combination of local and national priorities and conformed to a national framework of good practice. It would be the subject of wide local scrutiny and debate, with a strong preventive element and public health component. So, for example, while childhood obesity continues to grow, the CST plan would produce recommendations as to how it would be tackled at a local level. There would also be a particular emphasis on demonstrating, in the report, how these integrated services were particularly focused on early years. After all, if this is properly addressed, the need for subsequent intervention should be reduced. The shared assessment and referral framework, outlined above would also allow the interrogation of data, to look at emerging local trends, ensure the team was representing local priorities, measure progress against targets and submit data to be collected nationally, in order to make comparisons.

We can now test how far the principles of integration outlined by BACCH, in Chapter 6, are met by this integrated model. First, it is demonstrably child focused with a multi-disciplinary team able to respond holistically to a child's needs, through the medium of a Named Person who appropriately involves other services. Integration across the whole pathway of a child's life should be more possible, through an earlier access to other services. This, in turn, should lead to an improvement in the quality of care, measured partly by a robust information system, which not only tracks support and treatment but allows research into effectiveness. The introduction of a Local Management Board permits some real stakeholder engagement – a cornerstone of the BACCH principles – and allows decisions about how the pooled budget will be utilised. It is to be hoped that the co-location of staff will also allow the development of shared values and some adjustment as to how priorities for treatment and support are made; both at an individual level and across the total population of children and young people being served.

Lastly, BACCH rightly stresses the need for political support when any model of integration is being sought. The engagement of local politicians, through the local CST Management Boards, is crucial to the success of the CSTs if they are to be responsive to the needs of any community.

The Appendix provides examples of how, on an individual basis, an integrated model of child care can be seen to work. The often empty rhetoric of "wraparound services" or "the team around the child" are here replaced by examples of what real "joined up services" for children might look like.

In the case studies all of the children have tier 2–4 needs. Each requires services above and beyond those of the majority of the child population and would therefore be referred to the CST. In order to argue for a workable new model, it is essential to demonstrate both that it is robust and works across a wide spectrum of challenging circumstances. Inevitably, CSTs will take time to settle down. They are not a quick fix and the last element of their implementation needs to be an extensive action research programme. This will be aimed at concentrating on "what works", sharing good practice as the CSTs evolve and making those changes necessary to best serve the needs of children and families.

Notes

1 *Trends in consultation rates in general practice.* Health and Social Care Information Centre. Quoted in General Practice in the UK-background briefing. British Medical Association, 2017.
2 *Best practice for a Sure Start. The way forward for children's centres.* Report from the All Parliamentary Sure Start group. July 2013 published by 4Children.
3 *Every child matters.* The Treasury. CM5860, 2003, HMSO.
4 *Matching needs and services in the audit and planning of provision for children looked after by local authorities.* Dartington Social Research Unit, 1995, Dartington.

9

WHOSE CHILDREN?

"It is", as Alan Bennett has remarked, "a good job childhood is at the beginning of our lives. We'd never survive it if it were in the middle" (1). He was writing specifically of the indignities and disappointments John Betjeman experienced as a child and that sense of unfairness that many of us will recall. However, many children successfully negotiate their way through the experience, even with the increasing challenges of ever-rising educational expectations, economic pressures and the social media. But for those who don't, and require extra help and support, the book has argued that they often experience fractured and bifurcated services.

This lack of connectedness and separation of care begins right at the top of government. As Helen Seaford noted:

> The child moves through Whitehall growing and shrinking like Alice: in the Department of Health she is a small potential victim, at the Treasury and Department of Education a growing but silent unit of investment, but at the Home Office a huge and threatening yob.
>
> *(2, pp. 454–465)*

Even limited attempts at joining ministries have not proved sustainable, with, for example, the Department of Children, Schools and Families, bringing together education and social care in 2007 and affecting young people in England up to the age of 19, including child protection, and later to be dismantled with a change of government in 2010.

Not only is government not connected when it comes to the care of children but so, too, is the judiciary. In his Parmoor lecture, referred to in Chapter 3, Sir James Munby argued that there was a spread of responsibility across the courts.

When a child is to be put into the care of a local authority "and disputes in relation to what until recently were called residence and contact" (3, p. 6) these are heard in the Family Court or the Family Division of the High Court. However, criminal cases where a child is being prosecuted are held in the youth court or the Crown Court. Or where a child is seeking asylum or is subject to immigration control, the case is heard in the First-tier and Upper Tribunals of the Immigration and Asylum Chamber. Lastly, where a child is subject to the provisions of the Mental Health Act 1983, then here the relevant tribunal is the Health, Education and Social Care Chamber.

As Sir James Munby argues, while there are some mechanisms in place for sharing information there are no processes for joint or even joined up decision-making:

> I remember a case some years ago where both the family court and the Youth Court had made orders providing for the involvement of the relevant local authority in the child's life. The child lived in London; the family legislation decreed that the relevant authority was the London Borough of A, the criminal legislation that the relevant authority was the London Borough of B. Did the child benefit from having the services of two local authorities? The answer, as you may have guessed, was No. The involvement of two authorities was simply a recipe for confusion leading to inertia.
>
> *(3, p. 3)*

For Sir James Munby, all of this is compounded by two equally large problems: the wide divergence of those responsible for budgets and, to return to an earlier point, the disjointed division of responsibilities across Whitehall departments. He lists:

- The Department of Education
- The Ministry of Justice
- The Department of Health
- The Home Office
- The Department for Work and Pensions
- The Department for Communities and Local Government
- The Department for Digital, Culture, Media and Sport

as all having some government engagement in youthful lives but, as we saw in Chapter 3, no ministry with an overall responsibility for children and young people.

It is not surprising that we find the same divergence, duplication and separation of children's services at a local level. Ironically, as far back as 1945, Lady Allen of Hurtwood's evidence to the Curtis Committee (which, eventually led to the establishment of Children's Departments) argued that the responsibility for children could best be accepted and discharged by one government department:

> In my opinion the Department should be the Ministry of Education . . . There should, therefore, be created within the Department a special Division responsible for all aspects of the care of these children, including their health, their education, their aftercare and staff training.
>
> *(4, p. 2)*

And, almost as an afterthought, she added a footnote that still has a resonance today:

> One of the most unfortunate features of the present system is that the overlapping of departmental functions has made it difficult to regard the child as an individual who needs continuity of method and environment.
>
> *(4, p. 3)*

As we have seen, with this fragmentation has come the short-termism that seems to characterise policies for children, whether across health, social care or education. It would be little short of naïve to deny that, first, ministers partly make their reputations by the carousel of scrapping the projects of their predecessors and announcing policy initiatives of their own – whether the result of public pressures or ideology. Second, that political beliefs differ very widely within and between administrations. It is, however, tempting to ask the question as to whether other areas of government are subject to the same degree of hokey cokey policy making that demonstrably happens to children and young people.

It is also tempting to question whether this is worse in the UK than say, in other European countries. We saw in Chapter 4 that, according to the UNICEF report, the UK is falling behind on a number of significant childhood indices. We looked in some detail, too, at the RCPCH's 2017 *State of Child Health* report (5), which has been followed up and strengthened by subsequent research between the Nuffield Trust and RCPCH (6) that looked internationally at child health measures over time and across 14 comparable countries. A few examples from the research indicate that, in 2014, the UK had the fourth highest infant mortality rate among all comparable countries, the uptake of vaccines for conditions like diphtheria and tetanus lagged behind a number of other European countries and the UK has considerably more overweight or obese children than the average amongst high income countries. Admittedly, these are selective statistics, but we saw earlier in the book that according to other international criteria, the UK does not fare well across not only health but social care and education.

In education, for example, one of the boldest experiments that has taken place, since the 1944 Education Act – the establishment of multi academy trusts and "self-improving schools" – was, in 2018, assessed to be failing pupils in many significant respects. A survey of 700 head teachers and 47 schools across 4 localities between 2014 and 2017 was accompanied by the analysis of Ofsted results over a ten-year period, to explore whether reforms since 2010 represent a genuine basis for an equitable and inclusive "school-led system". It might be argued that the answering of this question strikes at the heart of any society striving for inclusion in its education provision. The major research conclusions, from an educational experiment introduced by a Labour government but then modified and pursued by the Conservatives, was that schools had become more tightly regulated. At the same time there was a relentless pressure on test outcomes; a "chaotic system of winners and losers" with success narrowly defined in terms of Ofsted grades. As a result, high-performing schools were accepting fewer disadvantaged pupils, so school autonomy was perpetuating inequality (7). It would certainly be the case that no government would seek these factors as the desired outcome of an inclusive education system.

We have traced attempts to provide what Lady Allen described as "continuity of method and environment", both nationally and locally in the UK and in some countries abroad. We also noted that there is not the tradition, in the UK, of a pedagogical approach, which automatically brings education and social care together both in the training of staff and the way that services are subsequently delivered. While the momentum for integrating health and social care services for adult or elderly care has grown considerably in the last few years, children's services have lagged behind. Partly this is the result of the greater complexity of children's services and partly by the way in which services are sometimes driven by local priorities. And yet the success of Multi-Agency Safeguarding Hubs indicates that for a specific area of children's services a considerable degree of integration is indeed possible. There are still considerable obstacles to overcome, not least that of an integrated database, accessed by a range of involved agencies and undoubtedly this would involve a considerable investment in new funding.

In fact, this investment in a shared database – alongside capital costs to identify the premises for CSTs – would be the largest cost of an integrated children's service system. The book explored the huge investment that is already made into children's services across health, education, social care and the voluntary sector, for example, without reaching a definitive view as to whether more is needed. But a shared service, with common budgets would, for the first time, allow some hard analysis of where costs are going, permit an end to much duplication and the potential to achieve real savings.

The point was earlier made in the book that we have little idea of the overall costs of a child whose life circumstances mean that he moves from, say, family centre to foster home, to residential care and – as is sadly sometimes the case for looked-after children – prison. No agency holds overall responsibility for what is spent, so no department is ultimately accountable.

Yet, if a more detailed analysis of an integrated children's service revealed that the existing gross budget spent on children across, say, health, social care, education, the voluntary sector was not sufficient, what greater use of national lottery funding could there be than establishing a world class service for children and young people? It could, for example, pay for a national network of CST hubs, each built to a high, consistent standard with surgeries, play rooms, interview suites, crèches and advice facilities.

Three major challenges faced the book from its outset. First, the need to avoid more disruptive re-organisation given the length of time such change inevitably takes. Social care, education and health services are battle scarred from re-organisations that consume vast amounts of energy and paralyse organisations, sometimes for years, as they are implemented while often demonstrating little tangible benefits. *Shaping Children's Services* is not just a sleight of hand, describing what is essentially a major re-organisation, but by another name. In the same way that staff in the Multi-Agency Safeguarding Hubs retain their professional identity while becoming part of a new multi-disciplinary team so, too, would the integrated CSTs operate. And what does seem to be grounds for optimism from the MASH teams is that emerging research evidence indicates that a new shared culture is born, which overrides that of any one professional group. This is a powerful argument. Through working together, professionals find a consensus over and above one narrower professional view.

The second issue – the length of time this model will take to implement – is undoubtedly the biggest challenge. Not only will it take longer than a single parliamentary cycle (and therefore risk being ditched by the next administration), but it would demand a degree of political consensus rarely seen in politics. It is for this reason that the book examined some relatively recent periods in history where change has not only been fundamental and large scale but where, as John Prescott expressed it in another context, tectonic plates have shifted – but also stayed shifted. Two of the book's examples – in the early twentieth century and during the 1940s – were such periods: both precipitated by war. And of these two the establishment of the Welfare State during and after the Second World War has the most to teach us.

Clement Attlee, the prime minister who oversaw the most fundamental social changes that the UK had experienced in the last one hundred years, had visited Washington in 1941 and been impressed by supporters of America's New Deal. He was keen to make an evolutionary leap in the idea of citizenship that would set Britain apart (8). He argued that we were able to organise for war and death and that we could also "be organised for peace and life if we have the will for it".

What this resulted in was a "cradle to grave" service that not only included health but also education, national insurance and family allowance. In terms of the establishment of the NHS, it meant the first comprehensive and free system of care, bringing together a previously tripartite system of voluntary hospitals (supported by private donations), health centres, (supported by local authorities) and GPs.

It was achieved by a parliamentary "post war consensus", which was hard fought for and went a considerable way to ensure that it lasted. It was undoubtedly aided by the unity that had largely existed between parties in the Second World War, but Atlee knew only too well that he would have to fight tenaciously to ensure, even with this background of unanimity, it would last.

An integrated children's service will need the same degree of inter-party support. It is a twenty year task, not achievable within the agenda of a single parliament. But given the argument in the book that services are currently failing children and young people, incremental change will never be enough. What is needed is the same vision, drive and shared good will that was exhibited in the darkest days of the Second World War.

The third challenge is implementing change of this importance and size in a climate where the world is turning in on itself, becoming more insular, protecting its own borders and responding solely to narrower domestic agendas. The vision outlined involves lifting eyes towards the horizon and doing what Attlee did, which is to plan for the future. But today's climate easily leads to eyes being focused on the feet.

Yet children and young people have never faced so much challenge – despite better healthcare, greater opportunities and more emphasis for some on their rights as equal citizens. Challenges centre around a cyber, on-line world where the implications of one new type of technology are scarcely absorbed before the next development comes along. Electronic borders have become permeable, so a child abused in Thailand can find awful pictures instantaneously on the net, sent via, say, Amsterdam to the UK and elsewhere. Controlling this and other forms of social media and Internet abuse, whether this is cyber bullying or pornography, is putting unprecedented pressures on children. And as the gap between rich and poor becomes more acute the dispossessed easily turn to drugs, violence and gangs.

For these reasons it is essential we build a first class, integrated child-care service that fully recognises the role of all the professions and fully engages them in looking holistically at the needs of children and young people. For, as Nelson Mandela said, in 1995: "There can be no keener revelation of a society's soul than the way it treats its children".

Notes

1 *Poetry in motion.* Bennett, A., 2002, Penguin Books, London.
2 *Children and childhood: perceptions and realities.* Seaford, H., 2001, *The Political Quarterly*, vol 72, issue 4, 454–465.
3 *Children across the justice system.* The 2017 Parmoor lecture to the Howard League for Penal Reform. Sir James Munby, October 2017.
4 *Whose children?* Memorandum of evidence submitted to the Care of Children Committee by Lady Allen of Hurtwood, June 1945.
5 *State of child health report.* Viner, R. (ed.), 2017, RCPCH, London.
6 *International comparisons of health and well being in early childhood.* Cheung, R., 2018, The Nuffield Trust in association with RCPCH, London.
7 *Hierarchy, markets and networks. Analysing the "self-improving school-led system" agenda in England and the implications for schools.* Greany, T. and Higham, R., 2018, UCL IOE Press, London.
8 *Citizen Clem.* Bew, J., 2016, Riverrun, London.

APPENDIX CASE STUDIES

The following case studies help to illustrate how the Children's Service Teams will operate. They are presented in the same format, with basic details about age, ethnicity, referral details, the allocated Named Person and the estimated duration of involvement. This would constitute Part 1 of the referral process, as outlined in Chapter 8. Supplementary information relating to a specific profession, such as medicine or education, would form Part 2 of the case notes. Clearly, the Part 1 referral form would require more information, such as addresses and other agencies that might already be involved with a child or her family etc. But, here, the format has been simplified – and a commentary added – to provide readers with some insight into the way the inter-agency CST would operate.

Harry is British, aged eight and in Year 4, Key Stage 2, at his local primary school. He tends to regard the benefits of education as overrated but has a good relationship with his class teacher. She has growing concerns about Harry and his behaviour during the previous term. He has been arriving at school consistently late, very tired, often hungry and complaining that he has had no breakfast.

His mother is separated but still sees her ex-husband who lives locally and is believed to be occasionally violent. Harry has previously confided in his teacher that he is afraid of his father when he visits. He has also told his teacher that his mother will have to give up their privately rented accommodation and find somewhere else to live. Harry's mother has also stopped her part-time cleaning job.

The class teacher has made a referral to the CST, via the education lead in the team. After an initial triage meeting, it is decided to allocate a social worker in the CST as Named Person. Because there are potential child protection issues, it is also decided to involve the police, alongside a part-time housing liaison worker, the GP, school nurse and benefits worker. There are questions as to whether Harry's mother is depressed and, given both the family's impending homelessness and low income, it seems wise to involve both housing and some income support assistance.

The agreed view is that this requires tier 2/3 engagement and the three domains upon which to focus are the "living situation", "family and social relationships" and "physical and mental health". There is the possibility of some voluntary sector engagement as Harry is a keen swimmer and referral to a local club is a possibility.

An initial assessment calculates between one and six months' engagement with Harry and his mother. Areas to concentrate upon include the family's housing, welfare benefits support and maintaining the good relationship with Harry and his class teacher. The GP may be able to offer support if Harry's mother is experiencing depression. While there are a wide range of agencies who can potentially assist, they would not necessarily have any direct engagement with Harry and his mother. They would take part in an initial discussion/case conference with the Named Person, offer advice and ensure their agencies were aware of the family's circumstances. This clearly applies to other cases outlined below.

Mia is British and one month old. After the usual heel prick test, shortly after her birth, Mia was referred for further sweat and genetic tests and diagnosed with cystic fibrosis (CF). Her parents are both very young and Mia is their first, much wanted, child. As well as the practical implications of looking after a child with CF, they are very unsure of the implications for future family life together. Mia and her parents are referred to the CST by their health visitor.

Initially, it is agreed that the community paediatrician will become the Named Person. Other CST full- and part-time team members who agree to become involved, if only in a consultative capacity, include the GP, health visitor, physiotherapist and social worker. There are no child protection issues. It is agreed that Mia should be recorded as tier 3 and the two domains of "physical and mental health" and "family and social relationships" need addressing.

There could be both voluntary and private sector support, as the locality has a support group for parents with children who have CF and the physiotherapy services are contracted to a private company. In terms of the duration of support, it will be ongoing but change with Mia's growth. The first six months will be intense, as Mia's parents are given guidance about drugs and starting the physiotherapy. They will also need genetic counselling from the community paediatrician about the possibility of future children having CF. As nursery and school provision comes onto the horizon for Mia, education will need to be involved to ease her transition into school and advise about additional support. It is expected that the CST will call an initial case conference, bringing together all of the professionals involved and fully including Mia's parents, so they can feel fully engaged from the outset. Most help for the family can be provided within the CST hub building.

Jessica is an only child, who lives in a prosperous part of the CST locality and attends a private school. She is British and 15 years old. Since Jessica moved schools at 11, her parents have been concerned by her increasing unwillingness to eat and her frequent throwaway comments that she felt herself to be "fat" and overweight. A year ago Jessica's parents promised to buy Jessica a horse, if she would increase her weight, which she initially did. But the weight gain has disappeared, and her parents are now seriously concerned she may have developed anorexia.

Jessica's parents refer themselves directly to the CST. The team allocate a clinical psychologist from the Children and Adolescent Mental Health service as the Named Person. In the locality this is a private service, which the CST has commissioned. A community paediatrician and the GP also provide additional support from the CST, via consultation with the Named Person. The education liaison officer on the CST can also make contact with Jessica's private school, if deemed helpful. Domains to be addressed are "physical and mental health", "family and social relationships" and "education and employment". Child protection issues will also be explored at the outset of work with Jessica and her family by the Named Person.

The CST set engagement at tier 3. There is a support group for carers of young people with anorexia in the next town, run by a voluntary organisation and a source of support for Jessica's parents. The duration of involvement is set at between two and six months, following a multi-disciplinary case conference including Jessica's parents. But anorexia is challenging, and the Named Person will hope that by intensive, fully engaged, support from the outset s/he can prevent the need for in-patient treatment and further weight loss.

Anik is four, Indian and son to Aisha and Dev. He has an older sister who is seven and very protective towards him. Anik has been diagnosed with autism and referred to the CST by a practice nurse, attached to the family's GP surgery.

One of the community paediatricians becomes the Named Person, with engagement from a CST social worker, speech and language therapist, GP and education liaison worker. Depending on the degree of Anik's autism, he is assessed at tier 2–3. Child protection issues will be explored and domains to be covered are "physical and mental health", "family and social relationships" and, shortly to be addressed, "education and employment".

Community health services are run by a private provider, commissioned by the CST, who offer speech and language support if needed. Anik and his family may be able to utilise a range of voluntary support. There is a funded Portage service for SEND children in the locality and a voluntary playgroup offers one morning a week for children with special needs (both, again, funded by the CST). There is also a local autism support group that Aisha and Dev could access. One of the large children's charities also runs a commissioned respite care service, which might be a useful resource when Anik is older. Aisha and Dev may in future require a night's break from Anik and a chance to spend time alone with their daughter.

The duration will be ongoing. Once the assessment of Anik's autism, speech and language difficulties have been assessed the Named Person may be transferred to a social worker in the team, to coordinate both education for Anik and also voluntary sector support, with the help of other CST colleagues. But most of the services can be provided within the hub, with a case conference involving not just CST key and part-time members but the full engagement of Aisha and Dev.

Jason is British, 15 years old and lives in council accommodation with his mother and younger step brother, Andy, aged eight. Jason has never known his father but is used to his mother having a succession of short-term partners. There is a suspicion that she may be involved in prostitution.

Jason has been in trouble with the police, received a youth caution and is now connected to the Youth Offending Team (YOT). The YOT make a referral to the CST, partly to raise concerns about Jason's brother, Andy, and his home life but partly to ensure clear lines of accountability between the YOT and CST. A youth offending officer from the YOT will remain the Named Person, but engagement with the CST will involve a social worker – to look at child protection issues – and education liaison both for Jason and his brother.

Jason is assessed as tier 2 with the domains of "family and social relationships", "social and anti-social behaviour" and "education and employment" to be considered. Estimated duration of involvement from the CST is one to six months.

In this situation the YOT retain primary responsibility for Jason, providing support and linking with other community resources such as leisure and sport. But links with the CST can address support for Andy, child protection issues and ensure that the family's needs are addressed holistically.

Jakub and Tina are both in their early thirties. They have five children from previous partners and a baby, Kylie (one year old) from their relationship. The five children's ages range from 4 to 12. Tina is Irish and her partner Polish. They have been together for two years.

The family are behind with their council rent and the housing officer has picked up that there are relationship difficulties between the parents. Aware that there are also six children in a three-bedroom house, the housing officer makes a referral to the CST.

A CST social worker becomes the Named Person. She convenes a case conference engaging the housing officer, education representatives from the children's schools and an income support officer. (Tina looks after the children full time and Jakub does some casual taxi driving.) Child protection issues, although not identified in the referral, will be considered as part of the assessment. Agreement is reached that this is tier 2 and domains to consider are "living situation", "family and social relationships"," education and employment".

Voluntary sector support may be available through the Home Start scheme, which operates in the CST locality and receives funding from it. This would potentially provide a volunteer to assist at home with the six children. Some relationship guidance provides another opportunity for the family.

It is hoped to provide some short-term intervention, to assist the family, lasting from one to six months. This would focus on the housing situation, benefits advice and liaison with the schools, to see if any extra support was required for the children.

Michael is an eight-year-old Caribbean boy, placed with Mr and Mrs Hamilton who are shortly to be his adoptive parents. He has had an unsettled life, was twice removed from his mother and lived with two sets of foster parents before a decision was made to free him for adoption. He has come to the Hamiltons from a period in a children's home, while suitable adoptive carers were found.

Michael was referred to the CST by the social worker from a voluntary adoption agency placing Michael. There are no child protection issues and a joint assessment by the CST places Michael at tier 3 with domains to be addressed being "family and social relationships" and "education and employment". The social worker placing Michael becomes the Named Person.

Other CST workers are a community paediatrician, the GP and school liaison officer from the CST, linking with Michael's new school. The duration of involvement is estimated to be between one and six months, although see below.

As a result of disruption to his life, Michael has missed key medical and dental checks. These will now be pursued by the community paediatrician with support from Michael's new GP. Michael's education has also been disrupted so an initial case conference, involving the social worker, Mr and Mrs Hamilton and other CST staff will also need to involve the school liaison worker. As well as Michael's new class teacher, the Special Educational Needs Coordinator may need to be engaged. Michael's integration into a new school will take careful and sensitive handling. The social worker may also consider a post adoption support group for Mr and Mrs Hamilton.

Since the challenges in older adoptions can occur after the initial settling in, "honeymoon" period, the possibility of re-opening engagement with Michael and his family will be kept in mind by the CST.

Lin is aged 18 and has a son, Matti, who is four months old. They are Chinese, with Lin living in the UK since she was three. Lin is bringing up her son alone, living in a high-rise council flat and quite isolated. There are few Chinese families living in the CST locality. Her boyfriend ceased all contact when Lin became pregnant and her family, who live over a hundred miles away, have virtually disowned their daughter.

Lin and Matti have been referred to the CST by a health visitor, concerned about their isolation. Lin has virtually stopped breastfeeding Matti, which the health visitor feels is a reflection of Lin's depression. The CST assess Lin and Matti as tier 2 and define the domains requiring attention as being "family and social relationships" and "physical and mental health".

The health visitor becomes the Named Person with the GP, community paediatrician and housing support worker part of Lin and Matti's support team. Voluntary sector help may be available through a local crèche and family centre. There is also the possibility of linking Lin to the local Home Start scheme. The CST assess involvement as lasting between one and four months.

The GP would assist with Lin's possible depression and through the health visitor, the intention would be to put her in touch with other young mothers.

INDEX

Made in the USA
Monee, IL
12 November 2026

1ba956e8-921e-41d1-916a-efcc1cca46afR01